The Role of Transcranial Doppler Sonography in the Management of Pediatric Hydrocephalus

Authored by Branislav Kolarovszki

Published in London, United Kingdom

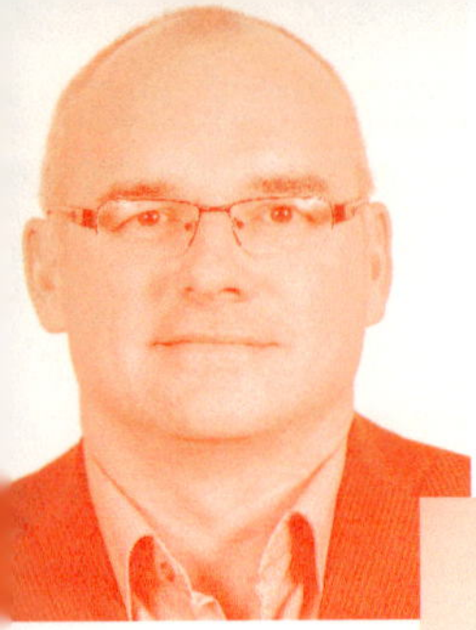
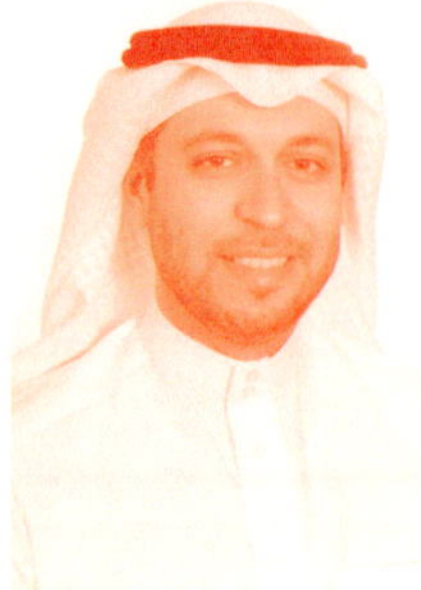
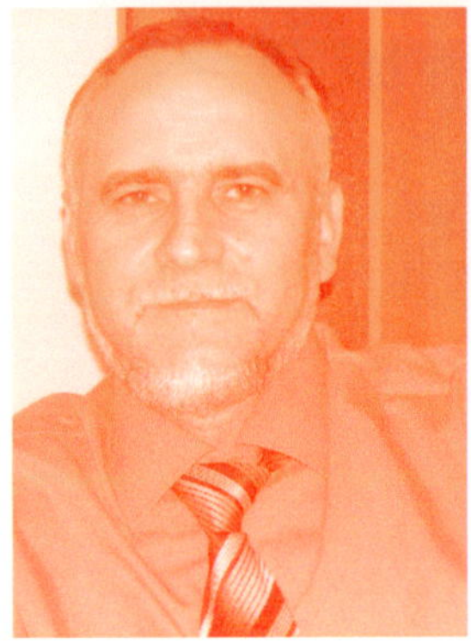
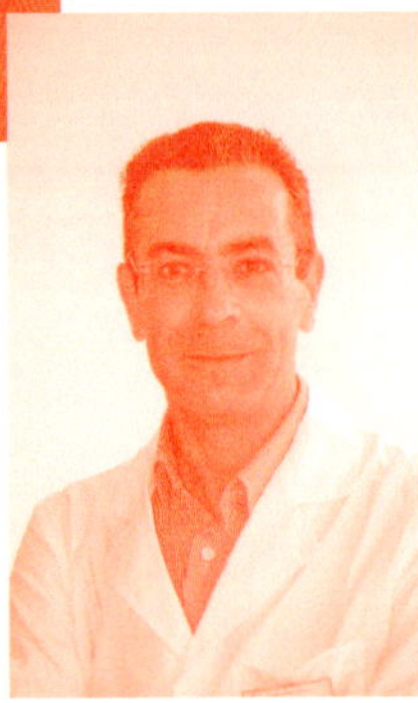
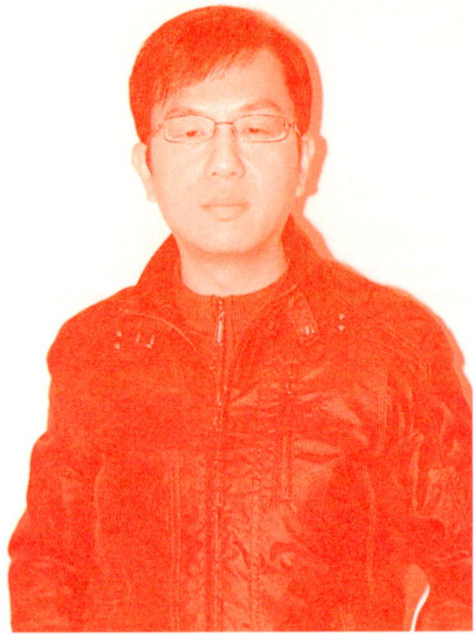
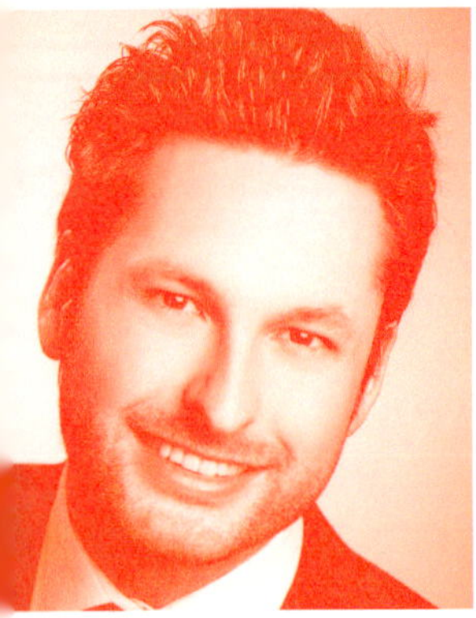
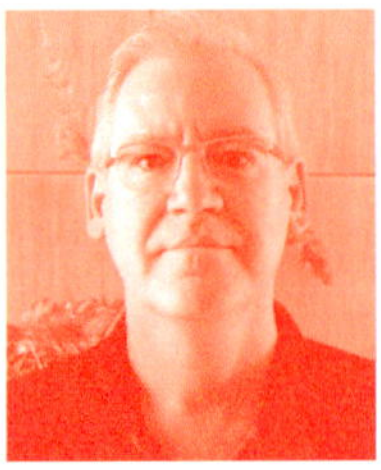

IntechOpen

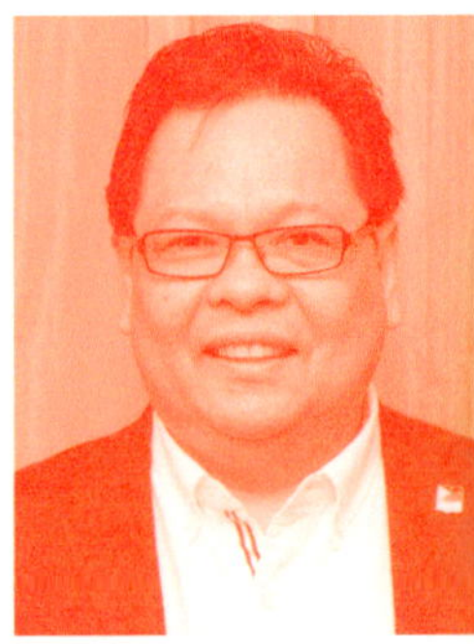
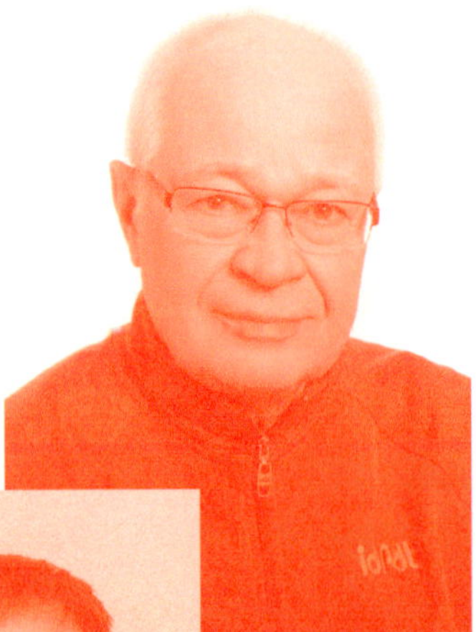
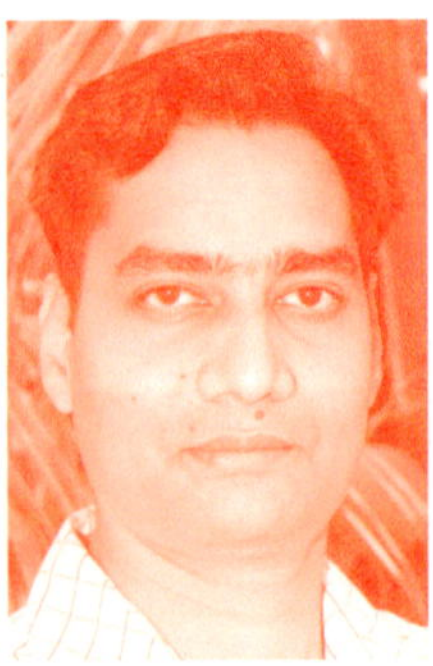
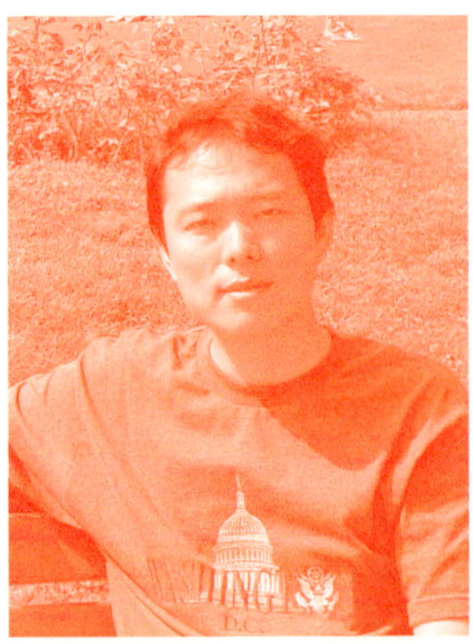
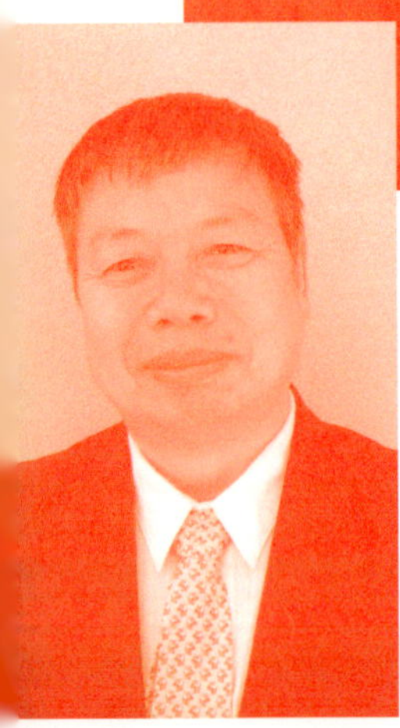
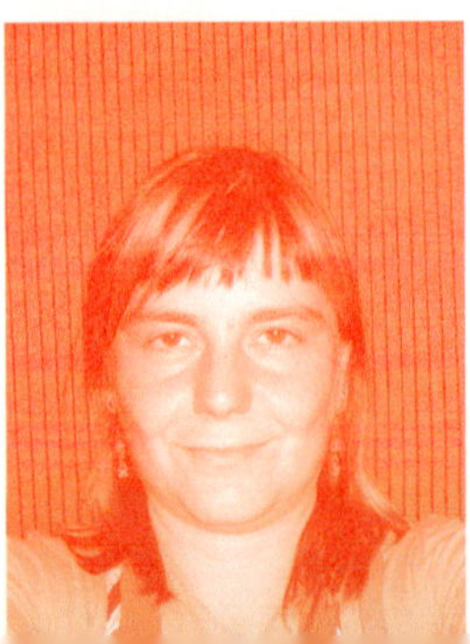

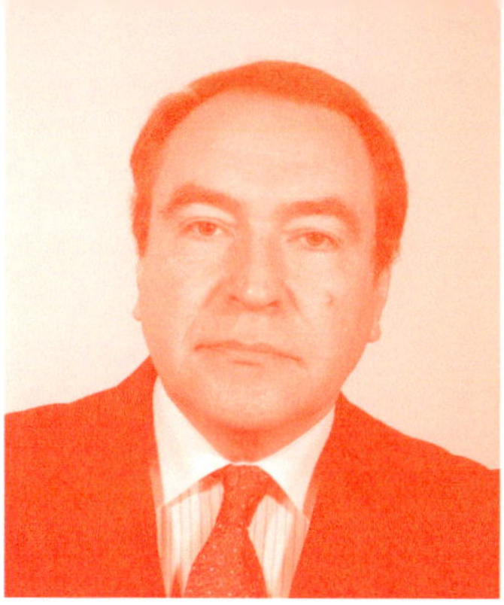
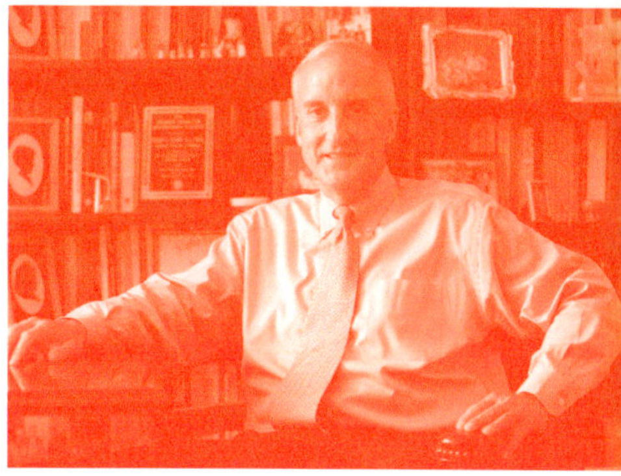
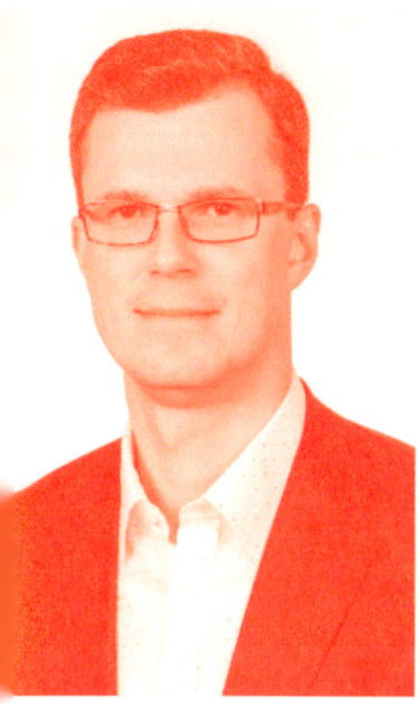
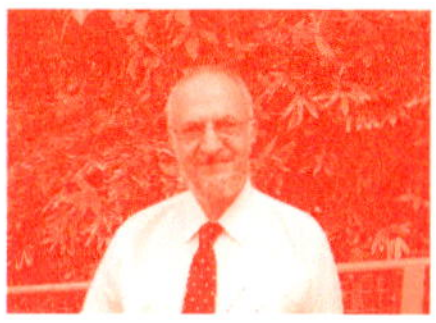
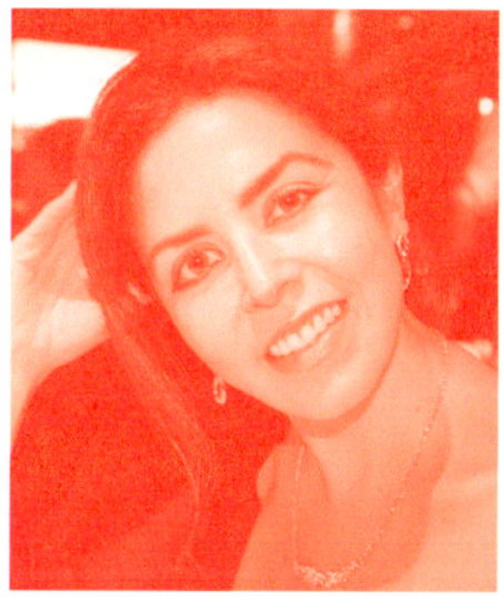

Supporting open minds since 2005

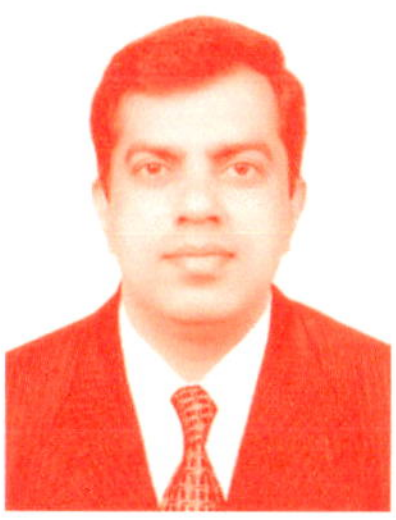
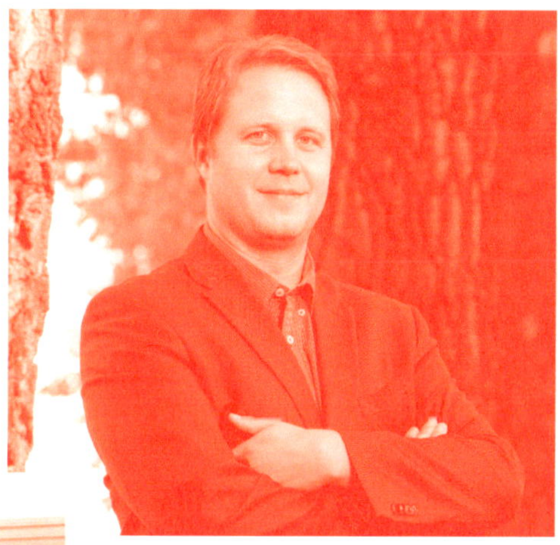
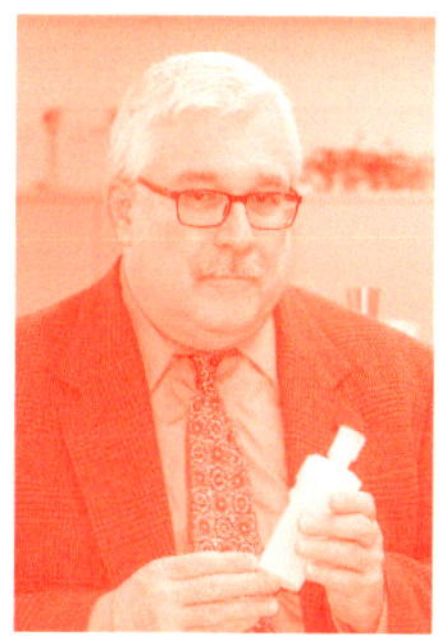
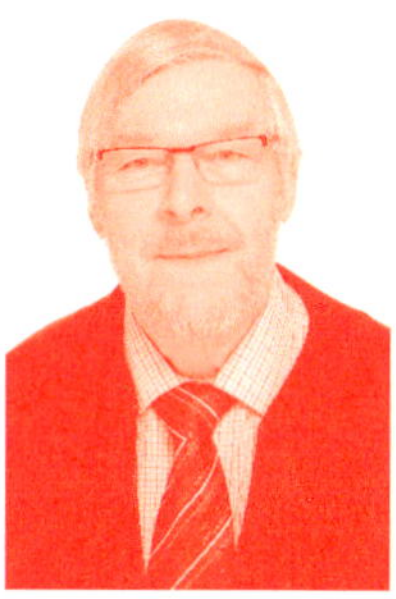
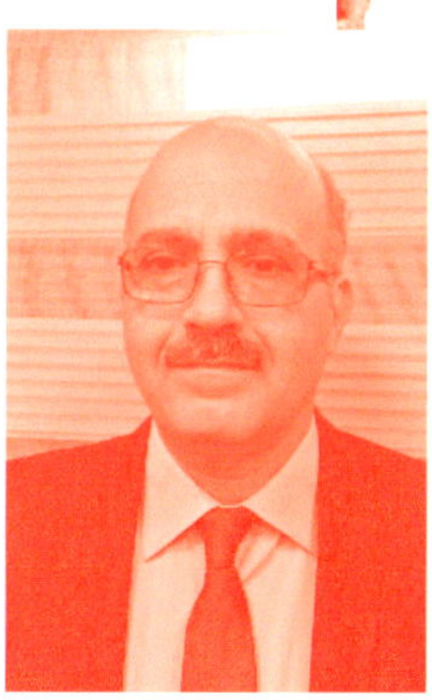
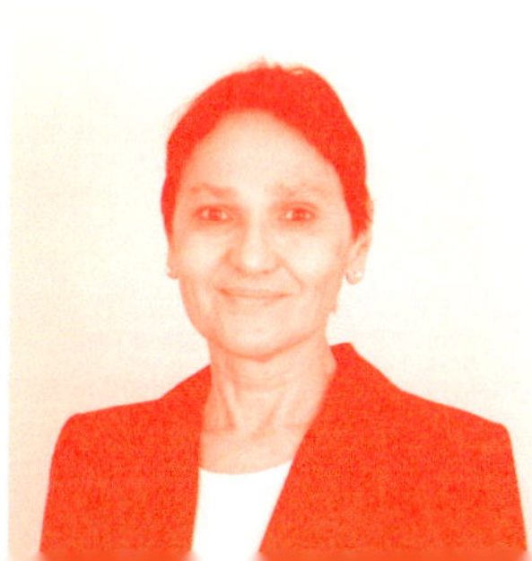
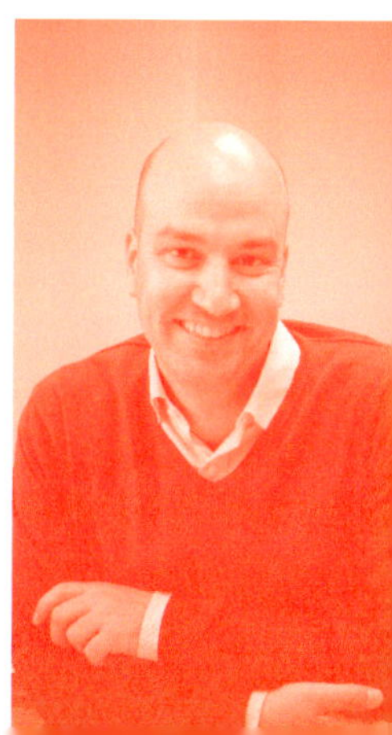

The Role of Transcranial Doppler Sonography in the Management of Pediatric Hydrocephalus
http://dx.doi.org/10.5772/intechopen.71092
Authored by Branislav Kolarovszki

First published in London, United Kingdom, 2019 by IntechOpen
IntechOpen is the global imprint of INTECHOPEN LIMITED, registered in England and Wales, registration number: 11086078, 7th floor, 10 Lower Thames Street, London, EC3R 6AF, United Kingdom
Printed in Croatia

British Library Cataloguing-in-Publication Data
A catalogue record for this book is available from the British Library

Additional hard and PDF copies can be obtained from orders@intechopen.com

The Role of Transcranial Doppler Sonography in the Management of Pediatric Hydrocephalus
Authored by Branislav Kolarovszki
p. cm.
Print ISBN 978-1-83962-444-5
Online ISBN 978-1-83962-445-2
eBook (PDF) ISBN 978-1-83962-446-9

For EU product safety concerns:
IN TECH d.o.o., Prolaz Marije Krucifikse Kozulić 3, 51000 Rijeka, Croatia, info@intechopen.com or visit our website at intechopen.com.

Meet the author

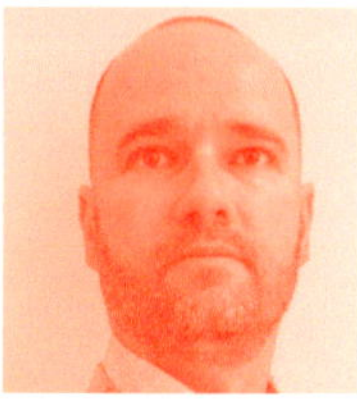

Assoc. Prof. Branislav Kolarovszki, MD, PhD, is the head of the Clinic of Neurosurgery, Jessenius Faculty of Medicine in Martin, Comenius University in Bratislava, University Hospital in Martin, Slovakia. He has dealt for many years with the issue of pediatric hydrocephalus and evaluation of cerebral circulation by means of Transcranial Doppler sonography in neonates and children with hydrocephalus. He published the results of his work in many scientific journals and two monographs. He actively participates in congresses, including invited lectures on pediatric hydrocephalus. Dr. Kolarovszki is a member of editorial boards and a reviewer of medical journals. He is currently the first Vice-Dean of Jessenius Faculty of Medicine in Martin, Comenius University in Bratislava.

Acknowledgements

This work was supported by the project on the application of picture archiving and communication system (PACS) in the research and development, ITMS 26210120004.

Contents

Preface

Recently, the pathophysiological changes that occur in children during development of hydrocephalus have been the center of attention. The current research is based on data gained in experimental and clinical studies. The amount of gained knowledge reflects wide scientific research. Extending knowledge about multifactorial-dependent brain damage in pediatric hydrocephalus allows changes in treatment procedures and improvement of functional results of the treatment.

Hydrocephalus is a pathological condition caused by excessive accumulation of cerebrospinal fluid, which leads to dilatation of the cerebral ventricles. Active, progressive hydrocephalus in children leads to increase of intracranial pressure, dilatation of the cerebral ventricles, and decrease of intracranial compliance. These changes lead to disorder of regulation of cerebral circulation and development of cerebral hypoperfusion, resulting in secondary brain damage. Ependymal disruption, periventricular edema, and compression of the periventricular capillaries can be developed. Ischemia of the white matter can be developed due to hypoperfusion. But it is reversible if treated early and adequately. In addition, there is damage of subcortical association pathways as well as decrease of the number of neurons.

Reasons for treatment of hydrocephalus in children by alternative drainage of the cerebrospinal fluid depend on progression of dilatation of the cerebral ventricles and manifestation of clinical signs of increased intracranial pressure. The dilatation of the cerebral ventricles itself detected by imaging methods is not an indication for drainage procedure. On the other hand, in the early stage, obstruction of the cerebrospinal fluid pathways does not have to lead to dilatation of the cerebral ventricles. But alteration of the cerebral circulation occurs. When increased intracranial pressure is present in children (in neonates and infants), clinical manifestations of the intracranial hypertension do not have to be obvious at first glance. Only part of them can be detected in the early phase, and thus it complicates indication and timing of the drainage procedure.

In 1982, Aaslid et al. presented transcranial Doppler sonography, which enables measurement of blood flow velocity in the cerebral arteries. Transcranial color-coded Doppler sonography, which has been used since the late 1980s, enables direct visualization of the cerebral arteries and clear view of blood flow in the artery. As transcranial Doppler sonography has been regarded to be noninvasive and appropriate for bedside treatment, it was also applied in children at any age.

Transcranial Doppler sonography enables to determine some hemodynamic parameters of cerebral circulation in various physiological and pathophysiological conditions. Qualitative and quantitative assessment of cerebral circulation using transcranial Doppler sonography is based on the Doppler curve. Interpreting changes in the cerebral arteries in the Doppler curve remains to be a discussed issue. Complex observation of intracranial dynamics in pediatric hydrocephalus, assessment of volume-pressure relationship, intracranial compliance, cerebral perfusion, as well as the use of knowledge in clinical practices has been in the spotlight. Generally, there is a good correlation between pulsatility index, resistance index of the cerebral arteries, and intracranial pressure. However, children with hydrocephalus represent a heterogeneous population, in which changes in the intracranial space need to be assessed according to various criteria, especially regarding age, stability of extracranial factors, and biomechanical compensation characteristics of the calva.

The complexity of relationship between the size of the cerebral ventricles, intracranial pressure, intracranial compliance, and Doppler parameters of cerebral circulation (when various intra- and extracranial factors influence cerebral circulation simultaneously) causes the measured values of Doppler parameters to not reflect the value of intracranial pressure in every case. This fact is one of the reasons why assessment of cerebral circulation using transcranial Doppler sonography in children with hydrocephalus is still discussed and an open topic.

This topic has been chosen because transcranial Doppler sonography is noninvasive and can be used in bedside treatment for indirect measurement of intracranial pressure and decrease of intracranial compliance by assessment of changes of cerebral circulation. The goal of this work was to assess changes of cerebral circulation in pediatric hydrocephalus and application of data from observation of intracranial dynamics in children with hydrocephalus in everyday clinical practice. The work is also focused on evaluation of impact of various intracranial factors on Doppler parameters of cerebral circulation, especially in neonates with hydrocephalus. The ambition of this work is to improve indication and timing of drainage procedure in children with hydrocephalus by application of the scientific results and clinical experience.

Branislav Kolarovszki, M.D., Ph.D.
Associate Professor,
Clinic of Neurosurgery,
Jessenius Faculty of Medicine in Martin,
Comenius University in Bratislava,
University Hospital Martin,
Slovakia

Reviewers:

Prof. Ľudovít Laca, M.D., Ph.D.
Prof. Mirko Zibolen, M.D., CSc.

The Role of Transcranial Doppler Sonography in the Management of Pediatric Hydrocephalus

Branislav Kolarovszki

Abstract

In the pathophysiology of pediatric hydrocephalus, a significant role is played by the negative influence of cerebral circulation with the emergence of cerebral hypoperfusion. Transcranial Doppler sonography is a noninvasive method that can be used for indirect measurement of intracranial pressure and decrease of intracranial compliance by assessment of changes of cerebral circulation. The goal of this work was to assess the cerebral circulation and intracranial dynamics in pediatric hydrocephalus. The work is also focused on evaluation of impact of various intracranial factors on Doppler parameters of cerebral circulation, especially in neonates with hydrocephalus. The ambition of this work is to improve indication and timing of drainage procedure in children with hydrocephalus by application of the scientific results and clinical experience.

Keywords: transcranial Doppler sonography, pediatric hydrocephalus

1. Physiology of the cerebrospinal fluid, cerebrospinal fluid pathways, and intracranial space

In physiological conditions, *the cerebrospinal fluid* is a clear, colorless liquid with a volumetric weight of 1007 kg/m^3 and pH value of 7.33–7.35. The list of functions of the cerebrospinal fluid is shown in **Figure 1**.

According to Archimedes' principle, the cerebrospinal fluid unweights and protects the central nervous system against a shock. This function is of great importance, especially regarding the fact that the brain, which weighs 1500 g, pushes on the base of the cranium by power of 50 g [1].

1.1 Production of the cerebrospinal fluid

In physiological conditions, 80% of the cerebrospinal fluid is produced in the choroid plexus in the lateral cerebral ventricles and in the fourth cerebral ventricle. The ultrastructure of epithelial cells in the choroid plexus corresponds with secretion elements. Cerebrospinal fluid production is an active process. Sodium-potassium adenosine triphosphatase (Na-K ATPase), which takes place in the atypical membrane of choroid epithelial cells, plays a key role in the cerebrospinal fluid production [2]. The choroid plexus produces the hemato-liquor barrier. Even in extreme conditions, the concentration of natrium, potassium, calcium, and chlorides in the cerebrospinal fluid remains the same [3, 4].

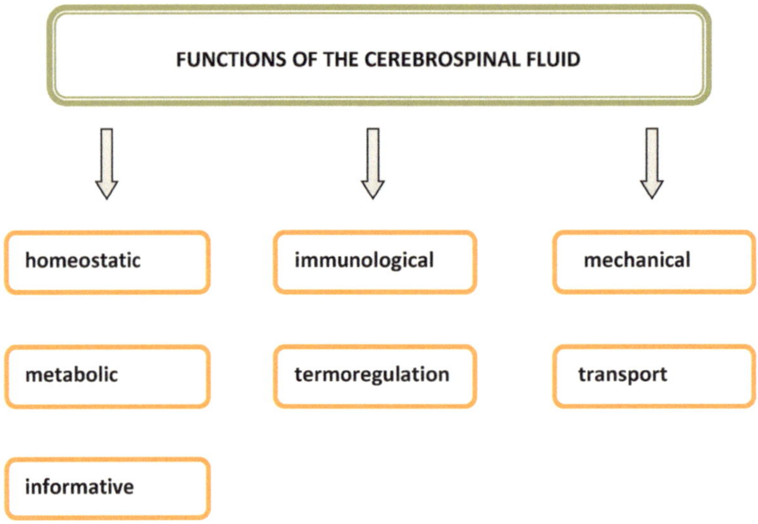

Figure 1.
A diagram of functions of the cerebrospinal fluid.

The cerebrospinal fluid secretion velocity is stable in physiological conditions. It depends on the weight of the choroid plexus. In adults, the liquor secretion velocity is approximately 21 ml/h [5] or 0.3–0.35 ml/min [6]. Daily, 450–600 ml of cerebrospinal fluid is produced, which means that the cerebrospinal fluid will change 3–4 times in 24 h.

The liquor production is not influenced by rapid changes of intracranial pressure in physiological range of values. Chronic increase of intracranial pressure, which occurs also in hydrocephalus, leads to atrophy of the choroid plexus and decrease of cerebrospinal fluid production [5].

Cerebrospinal fluid production can be influenced also by medication. The experimental studies confirmed that inhibition of carboanhydrase by acetazolamide decreases cerebrospinal fluid production to 50% [7]. The same effect was achieved when furosemide was administered [8].

The cerebrospinal fluid is produced also in other parts of the central nervous system. Most of the extrachoroidal cerebrospinal fluid is produced in the interstitial space and in the ependyma [5, 9]. The fluid gets into the liquor space via ependyma in the brain ventricles. Water and other substances penetrate in the subarachnoid space located in the cerebral convexity from the meningeal arteries and directly from the brain.

1.2 Cerebrospinal fluid circulation

Cerebrospinal fluid produced in the lateral cerebral ventricles flows through the *foramina interventriculares* (*Monroi*) into the third cerebral ventricle and through *aqueductus mesencephali* (*Sylvii*) into the fourth cerebral ventricle (**Figure 2**). From the fourth cerebral ventricle, it flows through *apertura mediana ventriculi quarti* (foramen Magendie) and *apertura lateralis ventriculi quarti* (foramina Luschka) into the subarachnoid space. Approximately, 80% of the cerebrospinal fluid flows through basal cisterns into the subarachnoid space of the cerebral convexity, and 20% flows into the spinal subarachnoid space [11]. From sinus venosus (superior sagittal sinus), the cerebrospinal fluid is absorbed into the venous system.

The circulation of cerebrospinal fluid is influenced by pressure of liquor secretion, ciliary activity, ependymal cells, arterial pulse waves, breathing, body movements, and pressure gradient between arachnoid villi and sinus venosus.

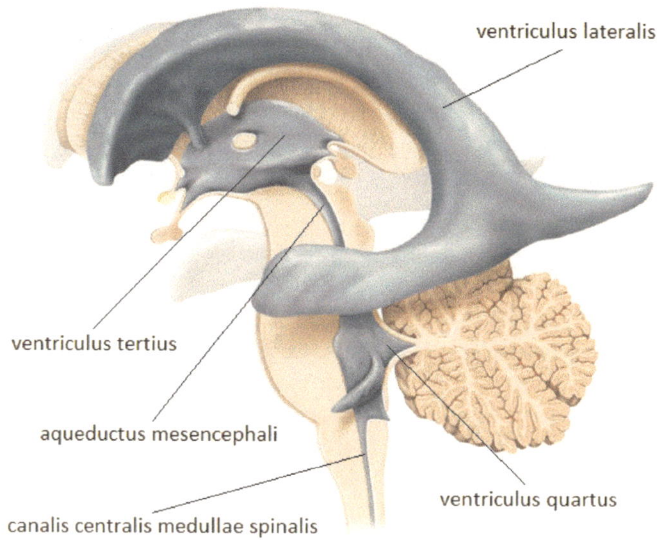

Figure 2.
The cerebral ventricles. Adapted from [10].

1.3 Absorption of the cerebrospinal fluid

Most of the cerebrospinal fluid is absorbed in arachnoid villi (villi arachnoidales). The villi protrude into dural sinuses and meningeal veins, at most parasagitally in cerebral convexity; a small number can be found in the cranial base and around spinal nerves roots. The arachnoid villi are one-way valves which enable cerebrospinal fluid to be absorbed into the venous circulation [11].

Inflow of the cerebrospinal fluid into the vascular system is a passive process based on pressure gradient between the subarachnoid space and the dural sinus. The accurate mechanism of cerebrospinal fluid absorption into the sinuses remains still disputable. Two contradictory theories about cerebrospinal fluid resorption (the process of filtration through membrane and direct flow of liquor in the arachnoid villi) were substituted by *the hypothesis of vacuole transport system* [12–15]. Rate resorption of the cerebrospinal fluid is pressure-based [16].

The cerebrospinal fluid is primarily absorbed in the arachnoid villi to superior sagittal sinus. However, there are also alternative ways for it to be absorbed. The results of some studies highlight the meaning of resorption through the lymphatic system [4]. The cerebrospinal fluid can be absorbed also along the cranial nerves and spinal nerve roots and in the *plexus choroideus* [6]. The exact meaning of the alternative ways of liquor resorption under physiological and pathological conditions is not still fully clarified. Some clinical results highlight a potential role of the central channel in the spinal cord in the cerebrospinal fluid resorption, especially in children [5].

1.4 The intracranial pressure

The intracranial pressure (ICP), defined as a hydrostatic pressure of the cerebrospinal fluid, is a result of active secretion, flow resistance, and passive liquor resorption into the venous system [5].

In the physiological range of values of intracranial pressure, the degree of cerebrospinal fluid resorption is the same as its production. The intracranial pressure is directly dependent on the venous pressure in venous sinus and then just follows its changes [17, 18].

In lying position in children and adults, the normal value of ICP is 12 ± 2 cm H_2O. In newborns and infants, the normal value of the intracranial pressure is lower. The intracranial hypertension in preterm newborns is defined as ICP ≥ 6 cm H_2O and in term neonates and infants as ICP ≥ 10 cm H_2O. The value of intracranial pressure gradually increases and stabilizes at the value of the adults when calvas ossificate and the cranial sutures and fontanelles close up.

1.5 The intracranial space

Monro [19] and Kellie [20] described the intracranial space as a closed compartment, known as *the Monro-Kellie hypothesis*. According to the hypothesis, the intracranial volume is constant, and the intracranial cavity is completely full. When the volume of any of the intracranial compartment increases, then the volume of another compartment has to decrease in order to keep the intracranial pressure stable. The Monro-Kellie hypothesis cannot be applied in all cases.

The exception is the cranium of neonates and infants before completion of ossification and closure of the cranial sutures and fontanelles. When volume of the cerebrospinal fluid and intracranial pressure rise (the cases of active hydrocephalus), then the volume of the cranium and the size of the skull increase, which leads to diastasis of cerebral sutures and bulging of fontanelles as a compensatory mechanism of intracranial hypertension (obr. 3–7). In any age group, the intracranial space cannot be considered a completely closed system because in the pressure-volume regulation, the cranial space communicates with the extracranial space through the carotid and vertebral arteries, jugular veins, and spinal cerebrospinal fluid compartment.

In physiological conditions, the intracranial volume is made up of 80% of brain tissue, 10% of cerebrospinal fluid, and 10% of intravascular blood. Volume of the brain tissue can vary because of the change in volume of cells and the change of volume of the intracellular fluid. The vascular system is connected to the extracranial space, compressible, and sensitive to fast changes of the intracranial volume. Extracellular fluid of the central nervous system is made up of the cerebrospinal fluid and extracellular (interstitial) fluid. They communicate with each other through ependymal lining of the cerebral ventricles and perivascular space.

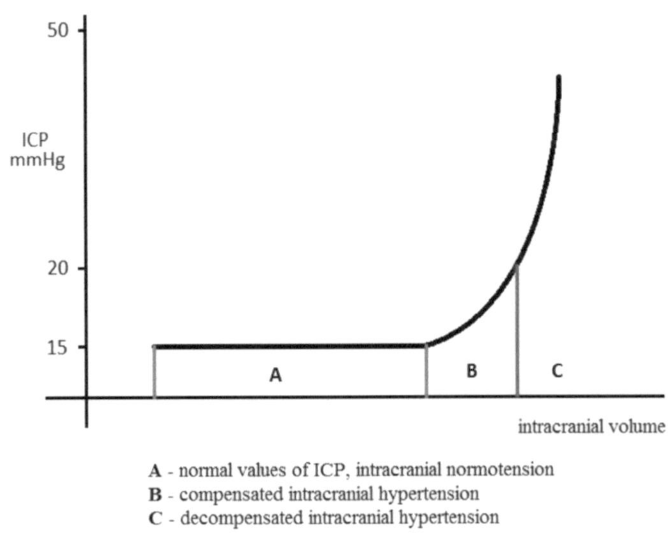

Figure 3.
The pressure-volume curve of the intracranial space.

The cranium of a newborn (preterm and term births), the cranium of an infant before and after the cranial suture closure and fontanelle closure, and the cranium of the children and adults have to be differentiated with respect to the intracranial dynamics. The dynamic characteristics of the cranium among newborns vary as well. The biomechanics of cranium is influenced by the size of fontanelles and distance between cranial sutures (in preterm neonates and hypotrophic neonates, the enlarged fontanelle and small cranial suture distention can occur). In infants, the fontanelles diminish gradually. Compensational distance of the cranial sutures in intracranial hypertension is limited, even impossible with higher age of an infant. After fontanelle and cranial suture closure, the child's skull gradually gets biomechanical characteristics of the skull of the adults [22].

Impact of volume changes in the cranial cavity on intracranial pressure depends on the condition of compensatory mechanisms (flow of cerebrospinal fluid to spinal compartment, decrease of blood volume in the brain, biomechanic characteristics of the skull and brain tissue). Tolerance of the intracranial space to accept higher volume without changes of the intracranial pressure is called *compliance*. Compliance (C) is defined by the relations $\Delta V/\Delta P$ (ΔV, change of volume; ΔP, change of pressure). According to the *pressure-volume curve*, when compensatory mechanisms are depleted, the value of intracranial pressure rises exponentially (**Figure 3**). When compliance is high, increase of relatively high volume may lead to only low increase of intracranial pressure. When compliance is low, small increase of volume is sufficient for significant rise of ICP. Elasticity is indirectly propositional to compliance ($\Delta P/\Delta V$). Elasticity is defined by the so-called pressure-volume index, which shows steepness of the pressure-volume curve [23].

Biomechanics of the intracranial space is influenced also by changes of biomechanical characteristics of the cerebrospinal fluid. Especially in the cases of infectious and posthemorrhagic hydrocephalus, the changes of rheological characteristics and liquor viscosity occur, which changes mechanical characteristics of the cerebrospinal fluid [24, 25].

2. Cerebral circulation

The vascular system of the brain is composed of the carotid and vertebrobasilar circulations. Both are interconnected by posterior communicating arteries (*arteriae communicantes posteriores cerebri*). The anterior communicating artery (*arteria communicans anterior cerebri*) connects both anterior cerebral arteries (*arteriae cerebri anteriores*). Despite the fact that blood flow in communicating arteries in physiological conditions is low, the arteries represent the main collateral connection between the intracranial cerebral arteries (*circulus Willisi*). The connection between the external and internal carotid systems is ensured by ophthalmic arteries. The connection between external carotid system and spinal arteries is ensured by occipital arteries. The external carotid arteries supply also the leptomeningeal arteries which may penetrate to the cerebral cortex. Symon [26] demonstrated effectivity of collateral circulation in the cerebral circulation in a monkey. In his work, he found out that complete occlusion of internal carotid artery resulted in 14% decrease of perfusion pressure in ipsilateral middle cerebral artery. When both carotid arteries were closed, the perfusion pressure in middle cerebral arteries dropped down to 50%.

2.1 Development of cerebral blood flow

Disruption of cerebral blood flow plays a key role in etiopathogenesis of perinatal and neonatal brain damage. Cerebral ischemia is considered as the main factor of damage of the cerebral cortex, deep gray matter structures, and periventricular white matter in preterm neonates [27–29]. Frequent consequence of the brain damage is disorder of psychomotor development and onset of spasticity [30].

From the 32nd to 42nd week of gestation, blood flow in the brain rises gradually. This is caused by simultaneous increase of weight of the brain and cerebral circulation. The cerebral perfusion reflects increased metabolic demand of the brain tissue when functional activity of the brain rises during fast growth and organization of the brain structures [31]. The rise of the metabolic demand of the brain during gestational age of the fetus was also confirmed in observation of glucose metabolism by positron emission tomography [32] and observation of the use of oxygen in the brain tissue by near-infrared spectroscopy [33].

A significant rise of cerebral blood flow (CBF) is related to increase of blood flow in the cerebral cortex in the next gestational weeks. Hüppi et al. [34] used 3D nuclear magnetic resonance and found out that proportional intracranial volume in the gray matter increased from about 39% in the 32nd week of gestation to the value of 52% in the 41st week of gestation. It is well known that perfusion of the brain gray matter is significantly higher than perfusion of the white matter of the brain. Blood flow in the cerebral cortex in neonates is about 10 times higher than blood flow in the subcortical white matter [35].

In neonates between 32nd and 42nd week of gestation, the relative involvement of the vertebrobasilar system in total cerebral blood flow is 26 ± 8%. It remains constant in this period [31]. Studies of various authors confirmed decrease of relative involvement of the posterior cerebral circulation in total cerebral blood flow from the value of 31% in 3-year-old children to the values of 24% in 18-year-old adolescents. The value of 24% has remained constant in adulthood [36, 37]. During observation of the cerebral blood flow circulation in neonatal period, childhood, and adulthood, no differences were found between genders neither in total CBF nor in relative involvement of the anterior and posterior cerebral circulation to total cerebral blood flow [31, 36, 38–40].

2.2 Blood flow dynamics of the vascular system

Particles moving in the lumen require force to transport themselves from one place to another. This force depends on pressure gradient between two points. Blood flow in the vessels depends on this phenomenon. Blood flow velocity is determined by two factors: pressure gradient between two points (force given by myocardial contractility and cardiac output) and the vascular wall resistance.

Blood flow velocity is directly dependent on a pressure gradient and indirectly dependent on the vascular wall resistance. Other factors, which have impact on blood flow velocity, are hydrostatic component (associated with gravitation), static component (associated with blood volume), blood viscosity, and diameter of the vessel.

In physiological conditions, blood flow in the vessels is laminar in its character. It means that layers of the blood flow move by constant velocity increasing from zero velocity value of the layer at the vascular wall up to maximum velocity in the middle of the lumen in the vessel. But the layers do not mix with each other.

When velocity of blood flow is high or the vascular lumen is narrow, laminar character of blood flow becomes *turbulent*. Critical velocity for onset turbulent circulation is defined by the *Reynolds number*, $Re = v.d.\rho/\tau$, in which v means blood flow velocity, d is the diameter of the vessel, ρ is the density of blood, and τ is the viscosity of blood. If the Reynolds number is higher than 2000, laminar blood flow becomes turbulent, in which the concentric and parallel layers of blood flow start to mix. This results in a number of separate flows with different velocity and direction to occur in the lumen of the vessel [41].

The blood vessels divide into smaller ones in various angles. In the site of division of the vessel, laminar blood flow becomes slightly turbulent. However, it usually is not important in terms of changing blood flow. Walls of the intracranial vessels differ from the walls of the vessels in the rest of the body in compliance and tension. The compliance of the intracranial vessels enables blood to flow in the vessels also during diastole. The cerebral vessels narrow toward peripheral circulation. If the cerebral vessel is narrowed significantly, velocity of blood flow increases in this place of the vessel.

3. Regulation of cerebral circulation

The brain has high metabolism of energy, approximately 20% of total usage of oxygen in the body. There is not any storage of oxygen in the brain. The brain cannot create its structural and functional integrity by anaerobic metabolism. It is an anaerobic organ. In these terms, it is necessary to ensure constant blood flow in the brain, which represents 15% of the myocardial output. Knowledge about regulation of cerebral circulation is needed for understanding of pathogenesis of various conditions (including hydrocephalus) and effect of medication to the central nervous system.

3.1 Humoral and metabolic regulation of cerebral circulation

Besides brain perfusion, it is also necessary to ensure relationship between blood flow through the brain (transport of nutrients and oxygen) and metabolic demands of the brain tissue. This relationship has not been fully described yet. However, when metabolism rises, in a couple of minutes, also blood flow in the brain rises [42]. Many chemical compounds, some of which are also metabolic products, play a key role in blood flow regulation in the brain (**Figure 4**).

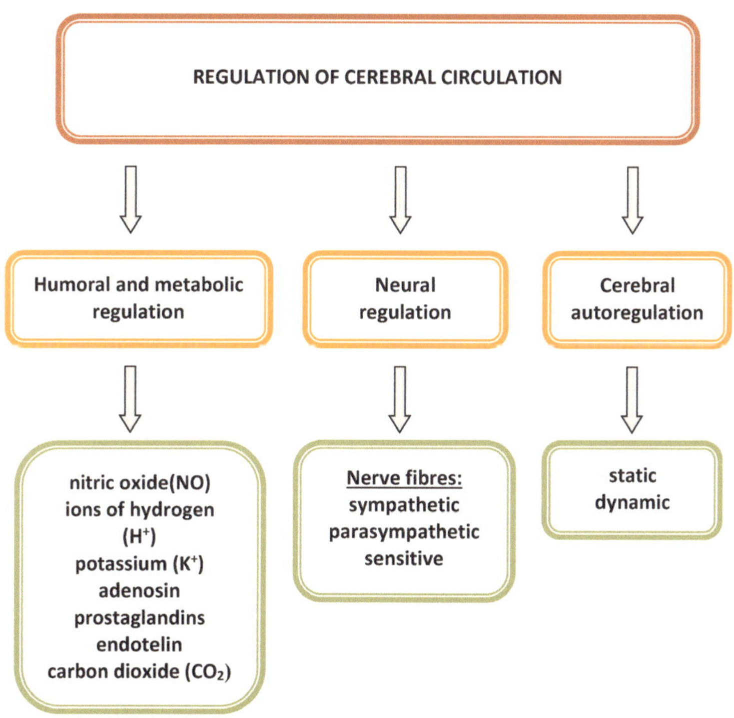

Figure 4.
Brief outline of the regulation of cerebral circulation.

3.1.1 Nitric oxide (NO)

Nitric oxide is catalyzed from L-arginine by NO synthase (NOS) enzyme. Three isoforms of NOS have been identified. Two of them are constitutive, present under the normal circumstances, and active, and one is inducible within a couple of hours (iNOS). Constitutive neuronal NOS (nNOS) can be found in neurons, astrocytes, and perivascular nerve fibers, while endothelial NOS (eNOS) is contained in the endothelium. Active NOS is calcium-dependent. Basal activity of the enzyme can be simulated by elevation of intracellular calcium concentration.

Both in in vitro and in vivo conditions, nitric oxide has a vasodilatational effect [43]. In the smooth muscle tissue of the vascular wall, it stimulates guanyl cyclase and increases the concentration of cGMP, which leads to relaxation of the vascular wall.

Decrease of blood flow in the brain during NOS inhibition is not related to changes in cerebral metabolism. However, it can be assumed that the release of NO during activation of neurons plays a crucial role in elevation of blood flow in the brain (Wang et al., 1993) [44].

Endogenous production of nitric oxide is related to the development and degree of intraventricular bleeding in preterm neonates. Increased concentration of NO with vasodilatation effects leads to increase of blood flow in the brain as well as to higher risk of bleeding in the germinal matrix, especially in sudden increase of arterial blood pressure [45].

Corticosteroids decrease production of nitric oxide [46]. It has been found out that in the antenatal use of corticosteroids, the preterm neonates have higher values of arterial blood pressure, need less vasoactive substances to support blood circulation, and are at a significantly lower risk of intraventricular bleeding [47, 48].

3.1.2 Hydrogen ions, pH

Hydrogen ions (H^+) are products of metabolism. Increased extracellular concentration of hydrogen ions decreases vascular resistance. The effect of pH change to cerebral circulation is of importance for response of cerebral vessels to carbon dioxide penetrating through hematoencephalic barrier into perivascular space, where it produces H^+ and thus changes pH value [49, 50]. However, in metabolic acidosis, hydrogen ions and other fixed acids cannot penetrate through the hematoencephalic barrier, so the resistance of cerebral vessels does not change.

3.1.3 Potassium

Increased concentration of potassium cations (K^+) in the perivascular space is caused by function of cell membranes. It results in dilatation of the arterioles with relatively low onset. In the cerebral vessels, there are several types of potassium channels such as ATP-sensitive channels and Ca^{2+}-dependent channels. When the channels open, potassium cations are released from the cell, and there is closure of tension-regulated calcium channels, resulting in decrease of intracellular concentration of calcium and vascular wall relaxation [51, 52].

3.1.4 Adenosine

Adenosine is a metabolic product with potential vasodilatation effect on the cerebral and the pial arteries. The velocity of changes of the arterial lumen influenced by adenosine is most likely too slow to cause fast changes in cerebral blood flow [53].

3.1.5 Prostaglandins

In the cerebral vessels, two isoforms of cyclooxygenase (COX-1 and COX-2) have been identified. Prostacyclin causes endothelium-independent relaxation of the cerebral vessels due to the activation of cAMP and K^+ channels. Indomethacin, an inhibitor of cyclooxygenase, decreases cerebral blood flow and reactivity to CO_2 and ICP, which may be accompanied by ischemic changes of the brain [54].

3.1.6 Endothelin

There are three isoforms: ET-1, ET-2, and ET-3. Under the normal conditions, ET-1 is produced in the endothelium of cerebral vessels. Endothelin causes significant and long-term vasoconstriction dependent on extracellular calcium concentration. In conditions when tension of the vascular wall was increased, decreased transcription of ET-1 gene was discovered [55, 56].

3.1.7 Reactivity and carbon dioxide

Carbon dioxide (CO_2) has significant impact on cerebral blood flow; the change in p_aCO_2 of 1 mmHg leads to change of CBF about 3–5%. Hypercapnia causes dilatation of the cerebral arteries, while hypocapnia leads to vasoconstriction. The relationship between p_aCO_2 and CBF is S-shaped with plateau below 25 mmHg and above 75 mmHg. Carbon dioxide has impact on the lumen of cerebral vessels by change of pH.

Many studies confirmed that carbon dioxide influences mainly the diameter of arterioles. When arterial blood pressure decreases, the autoregulation-related vasodilatation develops as a result of gradual decrease of reactivity to CO_2. In severe arterial hypotension (e.g., in neonates in critical conditions), vasoconstriction reaction to CO_2 may diminish completely [57, 58].

3.2 Neural regulation of cerebral circulation

Cerebral circulation, especially frontal circulation, is highly innervated by the sympathetic, parasympathetic, and sensitive nerve fibers [42, 59]. Sympathetic nerve fibers come out from the superior cervical ganglion, parasympathetic fibers from the sphenopalatine and otic ganglion, and sensitive fibers from the trigeminal ganglion.

The role of autonomous nerve control of cerebral circulation remains still controversial. Experimental studies on animals did not show constant change of cerebral blood flow under the condition of electric stimulation nor in autonomous denervation [60].

At the same time, impact of the innervations on relationship between CPP and CBF or response of the cerebral vessels to metabolic stimuli remained unclear [61]. New knowledge on regulation of cerebral circulation has allowed using transcranial Doppler sonography (Grubb et al., 1991; Diamant et al., 2002) [62–66]. Observation of blood flow velocity in the middle cerebral artery showed that vasoconstriction of cerebral arteries is connected to raised sympathetic activity during ortostase [63].

A study by Zhang et al. [66] confirmed that blockage of nerve ganglia leads to the alteration of dynamic and static autoregulation of cerebral circulation, which is accompanied by moderate but significant decrease of the cerebral blood flow. The authors assume that the autonomous nerve control of cerebral circulation is a tonic activity, which plays a key role in regulation of cerebral blood flow in beat-to-beat regulation.

It was confirmed that increased cerebral blood flow is due to stimulation of the ganglion sphenopalatinum. Despite this fact, the parasympathetic nerve control of cerebral circulation is not as clear as the sympathetic [67, 68].

3.3 Cerebral autoregulation

Cerebral autoregulation is a sensitive homeostatic mechanism, which is necessary for control of cerebral blood flow. In [69], it was defined by Lassen as an ability to sustain constant cerebral blood flow when perfusion pressure of the brain changes. This is called *classic definition of cerebral autoregulation*.

Experimental and clinical studies confirmed that the system of autoregulation allows to keep relatively constant CBF ranging from 50 to 170 mmHg (**Figure 5**) of the perfusion pressure [70, 71]. Mechanism of the autoregulation varies from relationship between blood flow and metabolism (coupling) and reactivity of the cerebral vessels to CO_2 [72].

The cerebral autoregulation is a complex of various physiological mechanisms, which differ in rate of onset and length of response. It can be assumed that restoration of CBF after an immediate change of CPP is due to change of vascular resistance in the cerebral arterioles [67]. In the restoration, two components play a role: fast response, which is sensitive to blood pulsation, and slow response, which is sensitive to changes of the mean arterial pressure [73, 74]. The responses are changing by activity of the sympathetic nervous system and vasomotor reactivity to CO_2. While increased sympathetic tonus and hypocapnia shift the range of the autoregulation to upper and lower limits, hypercapnia and vasodilatation substances decrease the autoregulatory limits [74]. In patients with chronic arterial hypertension, the autoregulation range is shifted toward upper limits of CPP [75, 76].

Alteration of the cerebral autoregulation occurs in various pathological conditions (brain injuries, subarachnoid hemorrhage, acute cerebral ischemia, intracerebral hemorrhage, and hydrocephalus) or is influenced by medication. In general, the cerebral autoregulation in the intravenous anesthesia is regarded to be intact. However, when inhalation anesthetics are used, the cerebral autoregulation is impaired [74, 77–79]. In the cases of the cerebral autoregulation impairment, even the small changes in the arterial blood pressure or CPP, if not controlled early and correctly, may lead to the cerebral hypoperfusion, development of cerebral ischemia, and edema [67]. The cerebral autoregulation impairment may be a sign of compensatory storage depletion of the cerebral circulation. It can be a sign of bad prognosis of the patient's condition [80–85].

When advantages of early *detection of the cerebral autoregulation impairment* were detected, there was a need for methods allowing repeated noninvasive bedside treatment of the cerebral circulation and autoregulation [86, 87]. Examination of the cerebral blood flow using xenon-133 clearance [88], positron emission

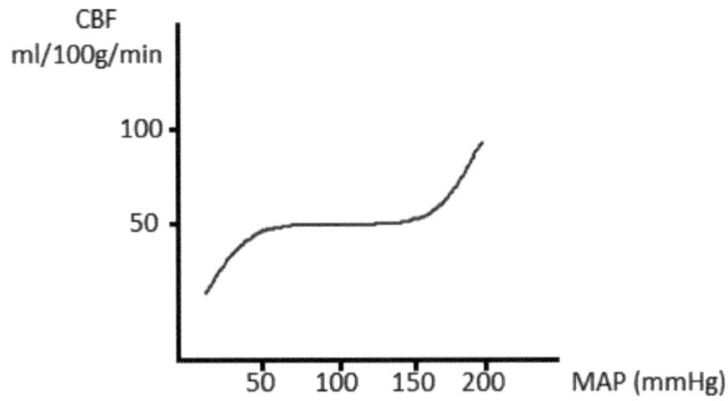

Figure 5.
Curve of the cerebral autoregulation.

tomography [89], and near-infrared spectroscopy [90] (Adcock et al., 1999) was technically and economically demanding and invasive. In general, it was clinically unusable, based on radionuclide methods including methodical and ethical limitations [31].

To observe the cerebral circulation, the transcranial Doppler sonography has been used successfully because it allows noninvasive bedside examination of the cerebral autoregulation by measuring the blood flow velocity in the cerebral vessels. Even though the use of the transcranial Doppler sonography doesn't measure the value of the cerebral blood flow directly, currently, it is widely accepted that the changes of blood flow velocity in the cerebral vessels in the fixed insonation angle reflect the change in the cerebral blood flow accurately [91]. Implementation of Doppler sonography into multimodal monitoring of patients with neurological impairment allows fast detection of hemodynamic changes in the brain and provides an opportunity for adequate and early change of the treatment [72, 92–99].

The cerebral autoregulation can be divided into static and dynamic. *The static autoregulation* describes a level of CBF change responding to CPP change in the stationary condition. It can be calculated by measuring change of blood flow before and after CPP change was induced. Normal static autoregulation response was described as a CBF change of 0.5–4.0% when CPP changed about 1 mmHg [64]. The next option is to calculate index of regulation (IOR) as a proportional change of CVR when CPP changes: IOR = %ΔCVR/%ΔCPP. Cerebral circulation resistance can be calculated using the following formula: CVR = CPP/CBF. If the proportional CVR change equals the CPP proportional change, CBF does not change. IOR value of 1.0 shows that autoregulation works well in comparison with IOR value of 0, denoting complete autoregulation failure [72]. Transcranial Doppler sonography has facilitated assessment of the static autoregulation by observation of blood flow velocity in the cerebral vessels [74, 79]. Then cerebral vessel resistance could be calculated using the following formula: CVR = MAP/CBF velocity [72].

The dynamic autoregulation defines velocity of CVR change when CPP changes in a certain period of time. The following formula is being used: %ΔCVR/%ΔCPP/time [72]. Most assessment methods of dynamic cerebral autoregulation are based on transcranial Doppler sonography [80, 100–105].

Dynamic cerebral autoregulation describes the speed of restoration of the velocity of blood flow (%/s) with respect to MAP change. The normal value of the dynamic cerebral autoregulation is 20% in the time to 5 s [64, 106].

Static cerebral autoregulation and dynamic cerebral autoregulation describe CBF change as a response to slow or fast CPP changes. Tiecks and Lam [105] described direct correlation between both mechanisms in patients with intact or pharmacologically impaired cerebral autoregulation.

Results of research confirmed that both types of autoregulation may be controlled by different mechanisms. Dynamic autoregulation is more sensitive to negative effects and can be impaired earlier than static autoregulation. Dawson and Panerai [107] confirmed that in acute cerebral ischemia, dynamic cerebral autoregulation was impaired, whereas static was intact.

Especially, neonates with the need of intensive care are sensitive to impairment of cerebral autoregulation [108]. Impaired dynamic cerebral autoregulation was detected in preterm neonates without signs of neurological disorders and in term neonates with neurological disorder. Both groups needed intensive medical care [109].

In [110], Lou was the first who described impaired cerebral autoregulation in preterm neonates detected by the xenon-133 clearance. Later Panerai et al. [111] confirmed impaired cerebral autoregulation under the dynamic conditions.

In normotensive preterm neonates, the intact cerebral autoregulation without reactivity to p_aCO_2 was detected. In hypotensive preterm neonates, the alteration or even failure of the cerebral autoregulation with decreased or no reactivity of CBF to

p_aCO_2 was detected [112]. Some authors found out that in preterm neonates, the cerebral blood flow is present even though there are low values of the arterial blood pressure. However, only static cerebral autoregulation was studied in these works [113].

3.4 The cerebral venous system

Approximately 15% of intracranial blood volume is contained in cerebral arteries and 15% in the dural sinuses. The largest volume of blood within the intracranial space can be found in the cerebral venous system [114].

The factors having impact on venous blood volume are as follows:

1. The vasoconstriction and vasodilatation factors
    - Neurogenic factors
    - Myogenic factors
    - Chemical and metabolic factors
2. Compression of cerebral veins
    - Volume of cerebrospinal fluid
    - Cerebral tissue (edema)
    - Tumors
    - Extravascular blood
3. Resistance of venous blood flow
    - Rotation of the neck
    - Obstruction of the jugular system
    - The head down position
    - Increased intrathoracic pressure
4. Cerebral perfusion pressure
    - Arterial blood pressure
    - Closure of the arteries

4. Definition and classification of hydrocephalus

4.1 Definition of hydrocephalus

Hydrocephalus is a pathological condition of excessive accumulation of cerebrospinal fluid in the intracranial space due to disorder of production and flow or

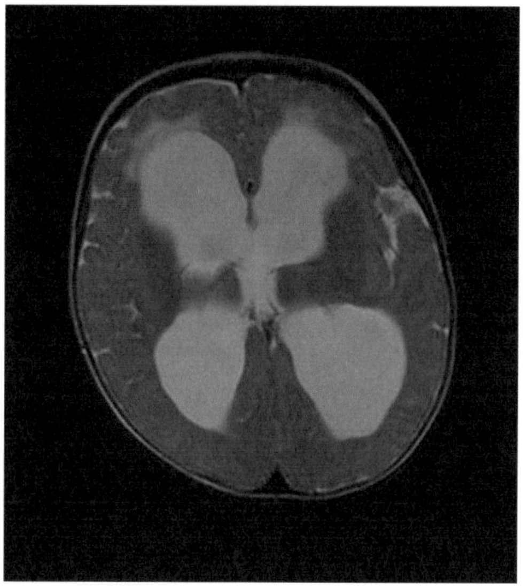

Figure 6.
The MR image of the brain (axial section, T2-weighted image) of a child with active hydrocephalus. Significant dilatation of the cerebral ventricles is presented. The finding of periventricular edema and roundness of the horns of lateral cerebral ventricles indicates the activity of hydrocephalus.

absorption of cerebrospinal fluid. Dilatation of the cerebral ventricles develops. In active hydrocephalus, it is accompanied by increased intracranial pressure (**Figure 6**).

In general, hydrocephalus is defined as a hydrodynamic disorder of cerebrospinal fluid, excluding hydrocephalus ex vacuo, in which the space developed due to atrophy of the cerebral tissue is filled with cerebrospinal fluid passively.

Prevalence of hydrocephalus is 1–1.5%, and incidence of congenital hydrocephalus is 0.9–1.8% cases per 1000 labors [6]. Incidence of neonatal hydrocephalus is dropping down because of decreased occurrence of congenital anomalies of the brain and spinal cord, which are related to hydrocephalus, and improvement of prenatal screening and postnatal intensive care.

4.2 Classification of hydrocephalus

Classification of hydrocephalus is shown in **Table 1**. Hydrocephalus can be divided into two functional types:

1. Obstructive (noncommunicating) hydrocephalus

    - A disorder of flow of cerebrospinal fluid proximal to villi arachnoidales (Pacchioni).
    - Dilatation of cerebral ventricles proximal to the blockage of flow of cerebrospinal fluid.
    - The obstruction can be intraventricular (internal hydrocephalus) or extraventricular (external hydrocephalus).

Functional classification	Obstructive (noncommunicating) hydrocephalus
	Communicating (nonobstructive) hydrocephalus
Types of hydrocephalus according to etiopathogenesis	Hyperproductive
	Obstructive
	Hyporesorptive
Types of hydrocephalus according to the course	Acute (days)
	Subacute (weeks)
	Chronic (months, years)
Types of hydrocephalus according to value of ICP	Hypertensive
	normotensive
Types of hydrocephalus according to the origin	Congenital
	• Hereditary
	• Acquired in the uterus
	Postnatal

Table 1.
Classification of hydrocephalus [22].

2. Communicating (nonobstructive) hydrocephalus

    • It can be caused by increased production of cerebrospinal fluid, decreased cerebrospinal fluid absorption (most of the cases), or insufficient venous drainage.

According to etiopathogenesis, hydrocephalus can be classified as:

1. Hyperproductive hydrocephalus

    • Overproduction of cerebrospinal fluid (in sporadic papilloma or hypertrophy of *plexus choroideus*)

2. Obstructive hydrocephalus

    • Obstruction of cerebrospinal fluid pathways

3. Hyporesorptive hydrocephalus

    • A disorder of absorption of cerebrospinal fluid

According to the course, hydrocephalus can be divided into:

1. Acute (days)
2. Subacute (weeks)
3. Chronic (months, years)

According to the relationship to intracranial pressure, we can distinguish:

1. Hypertensive hydrocephalus

    - Intracranial pressure is increased.

2. Normotensive hydrocephalus

    - Temporal increase of ICP values was observed in direct measurement of intracranial pressure. The value of intracranial pressure can vary and may be dependent on the relation to arterial or respiration cerebrospinal fluid pulsation [115].

Hydrocephalus can be divided into:

1. Congenital hydrocephalus

    a. Hereditary

    - For example, X chromosome-linked recessive hereditary hydrocephalus.

    b. Acquired during intrauterine development

    - Often called idiopathic because it is difficult to detect the cause clearly. In most of the cases, overcoming intrauterine infection is presumed but rarely confirmed.

2. Postnatal hydrocephalus

    - Hydrocephalus acquired after birth, during postnatal development.

Hydrocephalus ex vacuo. Dilatation of cerebrospinal fluid pathways is caused by atrophy of the brain tissue. Intracranial pressure is not increased. It usually occurs in adults because it is linked to higher age and neurodegenerative diseases (Alzheimer's disease, Creutzfeldt-Jakob disease, Binswanger's disease). It also occurs in children with neurodegenerative diseases and hypoxic-ischemic encephalopathy (e.g., perinatal asphyxia, posttraumatic conditions).

Hydrancephalus is a complete or significant loss of brain tissue. Occurrence of the small bundles of brain tissue corresponds with this diagnosis. Calva and meninges are intact, and intracranial cavity is filled with cerebrospinal fluid (**Figure 7**). The most common cause is bilateral hypoperfusion in the internal carotid arteries, which results in loss of brain tissue in the space supplied by ACA and MCA, while brain tissue in PCA is present. The other causes of hydrancephalus are congenital or neonatal herpetic infection or toxoplasmosis. Progressive dilatation of cerebral ventricles may imitate significant maximal hydrocephalus. These two types of hydrocephalus must be distinguished because re-expansion of brain tissue after drainage procedure may be expected only in maximal hydrocephalus.

External hydrocephalus is the enlargement of subarachnoid space in convexities of the cerebral hemispheres and basal cisterns in childhood. It is often accompanied with abnormal increase of head circumference, which is manifested with normal or slightly enlarged cerebral ventricles. *Idiopathic external hydrocephalus* (**Figure 8**) must be distinguished from symptomatic chronic extra-axial cerebrospinal fluid collections. Itis sometimes equated with benign subdural (extra-axial) collections in childhood. Idiopathic external hydrocephalus may be a variant of communicating

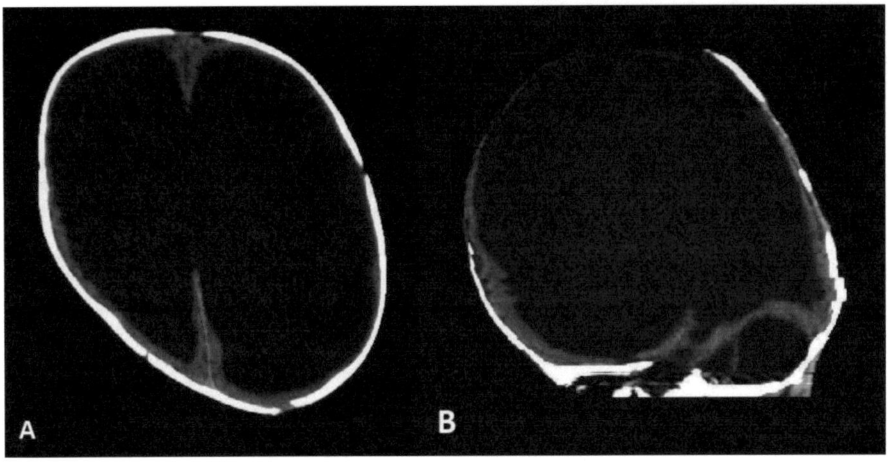

Figure 7.
The CT image of the infant with hydrancephalus. (A) the axial section; (B) the sagittal section.

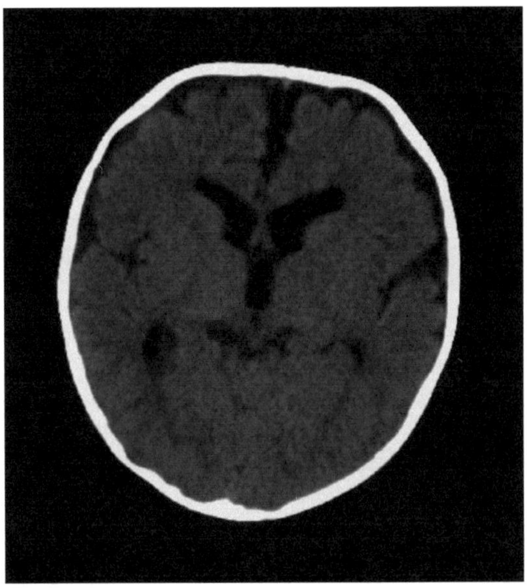

Figure 8.
The CT scan of the brain of the child with idiopathic external hydrocephalus (adequate psychomotor development of the child, no need for a drainage procedure).

hydrocephalus [116]. The cause is not clear. External hydrocephalus can also occur after intraventricular hemorrhage or obstruction of the superior vena cava.

The isolated fourth cerebral ventricle. The fourth cerebral ventricle does not communicate with the third cerebral ventricle through the *aqueductus* (*Sylvii*) or with the basal cisterns through the foramina Luschka and Magendie. It occurs in hydrocephalus with long-term insertion of drainage system in the lateral cerebral ventricle, especially in postinfectious hydrocephalus (mainly fungal) and in recurrent shunt infections. *Plexus choroideus* in the fourth cerebral ventricle carries on in production of cerebrospinal fluid. This leads to dilatation and increase of pressure in the fourth ventricle.

Arrested hydrocephalus is a term that has not been well defined and widely accepted yet. Some authors use the term *compensated hydrocephalus*. Most authors use this term to describe the condition, in which progression of dilatation of the cerebral ventricles or negative consequences of hydrocephalus do not occur. The criteria for arrested hydrocephalus without a drainage system are as follows [6]:

1. Almost normal size of the cerebral ventricles

2. Normal growth curve of head circumference

3. Appropriate psychomotor development

Stability of size of cerebral ventricles is determined by the use of alternative ways of cerebrospinal fluid absorption. The fragile stationary condition may be disrupted by various factors (fever, infection, mild brain injury), which leads to immediate decompensation of hydrocephalus with increasing intracranial pressure and need for a drainage procedure [117].

5. Etiology of hydrocephalus

Etiology of pediatric hydrocephalus is heterogeneous. Several etiological factors can determine development and course of hydrocephalus in a patient (**Table 2**). The causes of hydrocephalus are:

1. Increased production of cerebrospinal fluid

2. Disorder of flow of cerebrospinal fluid through CSF pathways

3. Decreased absorption of cerebrospinal fluid

Congenital hydrocephalus	Idiopathic congenital hydrocephalus
	Congenital stenosis of *aqueductus* (*Sylvii*)
	Chromosome X-linked hydrocephalus
	Dandy-Walker syndrome
	Arnold-Chiari malformation
	Postinfectious (intrauterine infection)
	Posthemorrhagic (intrauterine bleeding in germinal matrix)
	Caudal neural tube defects
Acquired postnatal hydrocephalus	Postinfectious hydrocephalus
	Posthemorrhagic hydrocephalus
	Expansive intracranial processes
	Postsurgical hydrocephalus
	Posttraumatic hydrocephalus
	Hydrocephalus related to spinal tumors
	Aneurysm *vena Galeni*
	Thrombosis of venous sinuses of the brain
	Achondroplasia, craniostenosis
	Hypervitaminosis A
	Constitutional ventriculomegaly

Table 2.
Etiology of hydrocephalus [22].

5.1 Congenital hydrocephalus

Idiopathic congenital hydrocephalus means that the cause is not clear.

Congenital stenosis of aqueductus mesencephali (*Sylvii*) causes 66% of congenital hydrocephalus. It represents 10% of all cases of neonatal hydrocephalus (**Figure 9**). In 75% of cases, the exact etiology of stenosis of aqueduct is not known. Stenosis of aqueduct can be primary or secondary. Atresia of aqueduct and division into several small channels, membrane composed of ependymal cells going through aqueduct, and aqueduct consisting of two blind-ended channels may be present. In a few cases, stenosis of aqueduct is present in hereditary X-linked hydrocephalus. In most cases, secondary congenital stenosis of aqueduct occurs due to gliosis after intrauterine neural infection or intraventricular hemorrhage.

Chromosome X-linked hydrocephalus (Bickers-Adams syndrome) is a gonosomal recessive hereditary form of hydrocephalus. Incidence is 17–36 cases per 1 million men. It is characterized by stenosis of aqueduct, severe mental retardation, and adduction-flection deformity of the thumbs, which occurs in 50% of the cases. Agenesis of the corpus callosum may occur as well.

Congenital postinfectious hydrocephalus, or an antenatal acquired postinfectious hydrocephalus, often develops due to intrauterine infection, e.g., toxoplasmosis (**Figures 10** and **11**).

Arnold-Chiari malformation. There are four types of them. Currently, only two of them are taken into consideration:

- *Type I*—a lower tentorial insertion; decreased volume of the posterior cranial fossa; a tongue-like extension of the cerebellar tonsils, which are moved to the upper part of the spinal channel; and attachment to the spinal cord. Hydromyelia and syringomyelia occur. But there is no meningomyelocele.

- *Type II*—the fourth cerebral ventricle is long and narrow, the cerebellar tonsils extend deeply into the spinal channel, and the medulla and the cranial part of the spine cord are extended and caudal.

In this respect, it is a kind of paradox that the roots of the cervical spinal cord go upward [118]. Myelomeningocele occurs in 90% of the cases and hydrocephalus in 70–80% (**Figure 12**).

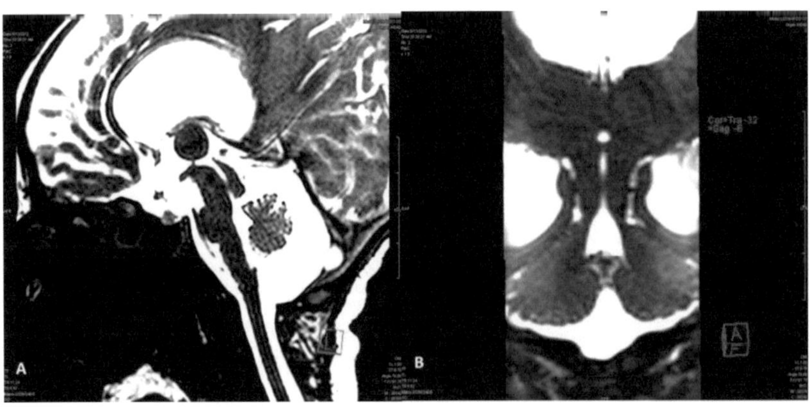

Figure 9.
The MR image of the brain (ultrathin sections focused on aqueduct) of the neonate with congenital three-ventricular hydrocephalus, finding of stenosis of aqueduct. (A) The sagittal section, (B) the coronal section.

DOI: http://dx.doi.org/10.5772/intechopen.89067

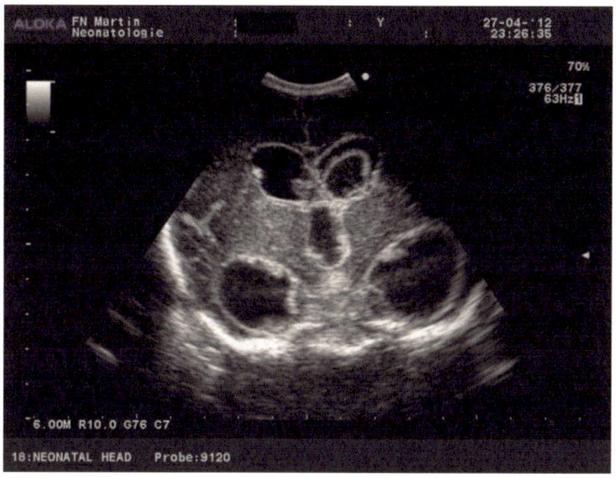

Figure 10.
The USG of the brain of preterm neonate after intrauterine toxoplasmosis. Postinfectious congenital hydrocephalus, the hyperechogenic wall of cerebral ventricles (the USG image of ventriculitis), hemorrhage in the cerebral ventricles, and hyperechogenic choroidal plexus.

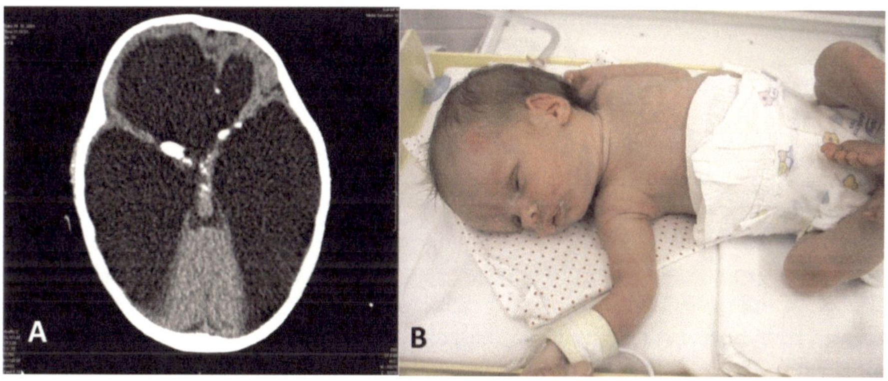

Figure 11.
The hypotrophic neonate with postinfectious hydrocephalus (after intrauterine toxoplasmosis). (A) The CT scan of the brain; calcifications and thin cortical mantle are present, (B) the photo of the neonate with the enlarged head, signs of asymmetric hypotrophy.

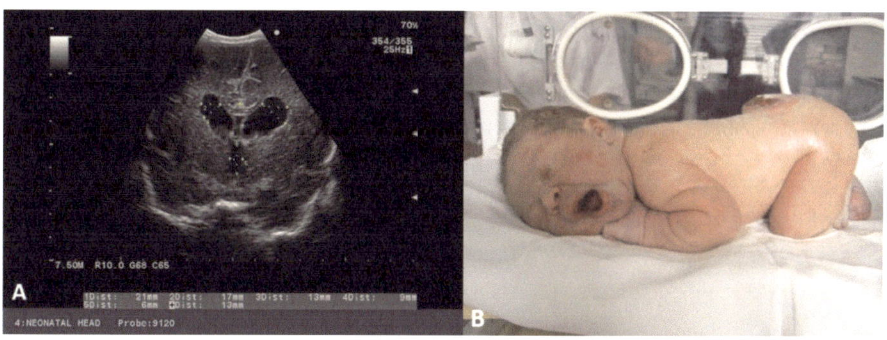

Figure 12.
The term neonate with Arnold-Chiari malformation type II. (A) The USG finding of the brain with hydrocephalus, (B) the photo of the neonate with lumbar sacral myelomeningocele.

Dandy-Walker malformation (DWM), also known as Dandy-Walker syndrome (DWS), is a maldevelopment of the vermis cerebelli, extension of the fourth cerebral ventricle, and enlargement of the posterior cranial fossa. DWM represents

5–10% of all cases of congenital hydrocephalus and 2–4% cases of pediatric hydrocephalus. The incidence is 1:25–30,000 born-alive babies. Girls are at a higher risk than boys. The exact etiology of DWS is not clear. The risk factors include chromosomal anomalies (3q+, 5p+, 6p+, 8p+, 8q+, 9p+, 17q+, triploidy), impact of isotretinoin in the first trimester of gestation, marriage between close family members (1.5%), and familial occurrence of autosomal recessive hereditary disease. DWM is characterized by six main signs: hydrocephalus, maldevelopment of the vermis cerebelli, cystic enlargement of the fourth cerebral ventricle, elevation of the transverse venous sinuses and their confluens sinuum and tentorium, increased volume of the posterior cranial fossa, and blockage of one or all orifices in the fourth cerebral ventricle [119]. In more than 70% of the cases, another anomaly of the CNS is present (agenesis of corpus callosum, stenosis of *aqueductus* (*Sylvii*), lymphoma in the posterior cranial fossa, syringomyelia, agyria, microgyria, heterotopy of the gray matter of the brain, defects of the neural tube, prosencephalon, colpoencephalon, infundibular hamartomas, occipital encephalocele or meningocele, hemangiomas, dermoid cysts, anomalies of the cores, and pathways of the brain stem). In 20–30% of cases, anomalies of other organs (macrocephaly, blepharoptosis, dysgenesis of the retina, choroidal coloboma, cleft lip and cleft palate, congenital heart defects, polycystic kidneys, polydactyly, syndactyly, anomalies of the lumbar vertebrae) are present.

5.2 Acquired postnatal hydrocephalus

Postinfectious hydrocephalus is mostly caused by purulent ventriculitis, meningitis, or meningoencephalitis. There is obstruction of basal cisterns and moderate dilatation of the cerebral ventricles, which may diminish spontaneously or prograde to active hydrocephalus, in which a drainage is necessary. Hydrocephalus ex vacuo may develop, too. Basilar meningitis may be caused by tuberculous infection. Blockage of the pores of Pacchionian granulations by proteins in neural infection may lead to hyporesorptive hydrocephalus. Neurocysticercosis is a common cause of postinfectious hydrocephalus in Asian countries.

Posthemorrhagic hydrocephalus is one of the most common causes of pediatric hydrocephalus (**Figures 13** and **14**). It may occur due to subarachnoidal hemorrhage or intraventricular hemorrhage. Hydrocephalus may result from obstruction of CSF pathways by blood clots or decreased cerebrospinal fluid absorption in Pacchionian granulations due to their blockage by erythrocytes and waste products after erythrocytolysis. Germinal matrix hemorrhage and intraventricular hemorrhage develop in 50–60% of preterm neonates who weigh less than 1500 g. Hydrocephalus may occur temporarily after intraventricular hemorrhage. Chronic hydrocephalus dependent on a drainage system develops in 20–50% of neonates with severe intraventricular hemorrhage [6].

Expansive intracranial processes can be benign or malignant. The most common causes of obstruction of CSF pathways are:

- Medulloblastoma
- Astrocytoma
- Craniopharyngioma
- Cysts
- Abscesses

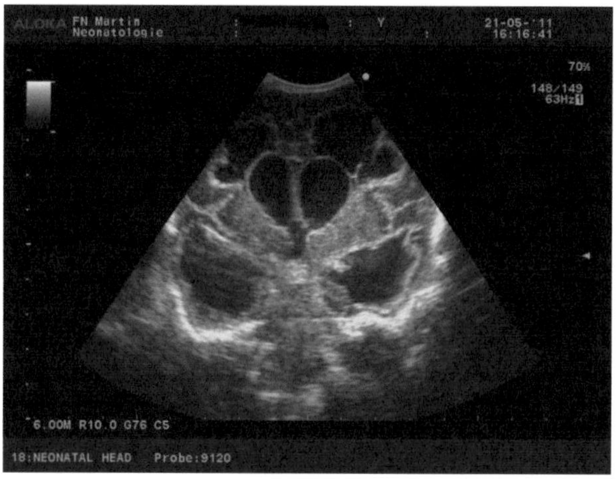

Figure 13.
The USG of the brain of the preterm neonate with posthemorrhagic hydrocephalus and multiple periventricular cysts.

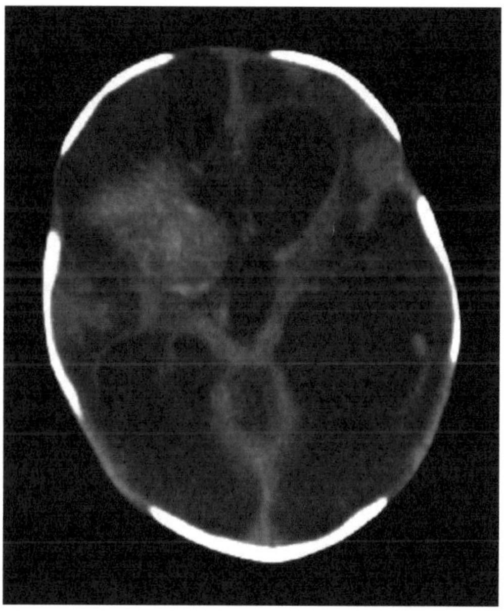

Figure 14.
The CT scan of the brain of the preterm neonate with posthemorrhagic hydrocephalus with diffuse hypoxic-ischemic brain injury.

Obstructive hydrocephalus in children develops due to tumors located in the midline of the posterior cranial fossa, the suprasellar area, the third cerebral ventricle, and the area of pineal gland. The suprasellar expansion of tumors of the pituitary gland or the expansion due to pituitary apoplexy may result in hydrocephalus as well.

Postsurgical hydrocephalus develops in 20% of children after tumor removal in the posterior cranial fossa. A drainage is necessary. Hydrocephalus may occur even 1 year after surgery.

Posttraumatic hydrocephalus may be caused by obstruction of CSF pathways in intraventricular hemorrhage, by negative impact on subarachnoid CSF pathways, and by resorption of cerebrospinal fluid in posttraumatic subarachnoid hemorrhage. Hydrocephalus ex vacuo may develop due to atrophy of the brain tissue resulting from a severe brain injury.

The cause of *hydrocephalus associated with spinal tumors* is not clear. It is assumed that increased concentration of proteins, increased venous pressure, or bleeding plays a role.

Aneurysm vena magna Galeni. Pathophysiology of hydrocephalus includes compression of *aqueductus* (*Sylvii*) by aneurysmal sac of *vena magna Galeni* and increase of venous pressure resulting from the arteriovenous shunt. This leads to decreased absorption of cerebrospinal fluid. Signs of heart failure are common in clinical findings in neonates. Hydrocephalus manifests later.

Thrombosis of venous sinuses of the brain may lead to the development of hydrocephalus. *Optic hydrocephalus* is an infection in the middle ear, resulting in the development of sigmoid or petrous sinus thrombosis. Thrombosis of superior sagittal sinus may develop if infection spreads directly to the sinus, in cases of severe hypernatremic dehydration and other thrombophilic conditions. Progressive communicating hydrocephalus may be caused by thrombosis of superior vena cava due to compression by tumors of mediastinum or long-term insertion of the central venous catheter.

Increased venous pressure in the venous sinuses of the brain may also occur in *achondroplasia* or *craniostenosis*.

Hypervitaminosis A may lead to hydrocephalus because of increased production of cerebrospinal fluid and increased permeability of hematoencephalic barrier.

Constitutional ventriculomegaly is asymptomatic and treatment is not necessary.

6. Pathophysiology of hydrocephalus

Currently, the main interest in pathophysiology of pediatric hydrocephalus is hydrodynamic, vascular, biochemical, and metabolic changes of the brain (**Table 3**). Deeper knowledge on multifactorial-dependent brain damage in hydrocephalus allows to change treatment procedures and improves functional result of treatment in children with hydrocephalus [120–125] (Williams et al., 2007).

The international congress *National Institutes of Health (NIH)-sponsored workshop Hydrocephalus: Myths, New Facts, and Clear Directions*, in which well-known experts on pediatric and adult hydrocephalus participated, was held from September 29 to October 1, 2005, in Bethesda, Maryland. The goal was to define current state and make strategy for further research of hydrocephalus (**Figures 15** and **16**)

Pathologic changes	Flattening and damage of ciliary apparatus of ependymal cells of the cerebral ventricles, disruption of ependymal basal membrane, diminishing and stretching of the cortical mantel, edema of the periventricular white matter, axon degeneration (demyelination), decrease of neurons, cerebral atrophy, perforation of septum pellucidum, compression of cerebellum hemispheres, and erosion on their surface
Vascular changes	Distortion of the cerebral vessels, collapse of capillaries, disorder of regulation of the cerebral circulation, hypoperfusion, ischemic brain injury
Biochemical changes	The role of neuronal death, Ca^{2+}-activated proteolytic processes, lipid peroxidation, alteration of neurotransmitter systems
Changes of cerebral metabolism	Alteration of energetic metabolism, acidosis, increased lactate concentration, changes in total volume of water, free and bound water in the brain tissue

Table 3.
A brief overview of pathologic, vascular, biochemical, and metabolic changes during onset and development of pediatric hydrocephalus [22].

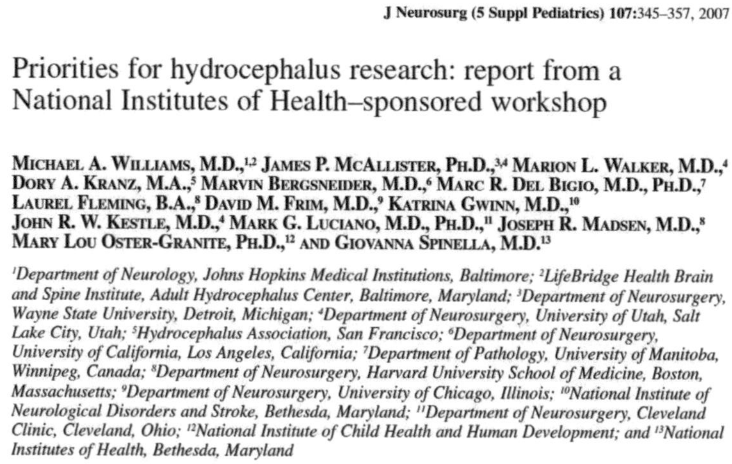

J Neurosurg (5 Suppl Pediatrics) 107:345–357, 2007

Priorities for hydrocephalus research: report from a National Institutes of Health–sponsored workshop

MICHAEL A. WILLIAMS, M.D.,[1,2] JAMES P. MCALLISTER, PH.D.,[3,4] MARION L. WALKER, M.D.,[4] DORY A. KRANZ, M.A.,[5] MARVIN BERGSNEIDER, M.D.,[6] MARC R. DEL BIGIO, M.D., PH.D.,[7] LAUREL FLEMING, B.A.,[8] DAVID M. FRIM, M.D.,[9] KATRINA GWINN, M.D.,[10] JOHN R. W. KESTLE, M.D.,[4] MARK G. LUCIANO, M.D., PH.D.,[11] JOSEPH R. MADSEN, M.D.,[8] MARY LOU OSTER-GRANITE, PH.D.,[12] AND GIOVANNA SPINELLA, M.D.[13]

[1]Department of Neurology, Johns Hopkins Medical Institutions, Baltimore; [2]LifeBridge Health Brain and Spine Institute, Adult Hydrocephalus Center, Baltimore, Maryland; [3]Department of Neurosurgery, Wayne State University, Detroit, Michigan; [4]Department of Neurosurgery, University of Utah, Salt Lake City, Utah; [5]Hydrocephalus Association, San Francisco; [6]Department of Neurosurgery, University of California, Los Angeles, California; [7]Department of Pathology, University of Manitoba, Winnipeg, Canada; [8]Department of Neurosurgery, Harvard University School of Medicine, Boston, Massachusetts; [9]Department of Neurosurgery, University of Chicago, Illinois; [10]National Institute of Neurological Disorders and Stroke, Bethesda, Maryland; [11]Department of Neurosurgery, Cleveland Clinic, Cleveland, Ohio; [12]National Institute of Child Health and Human Development; and [13]National Institutes of Health, Bethesda, Maryland

Figure 15.
The bibliography note on the title page of the publication by Williams et al. (2007).

(Williams et al., 2007). Research focused on pediatric hydrocephalus at our workplace follows the outcomes of this scientific event.

6.1 Pathophysiological mechanisms of onset and development of hydrocephalus

Mechanism of dilatation of the cerebral ventricles in hydrocephalus development has not been fully described yet. Dilatation of the cerebral ventricles is more than just a result of excessive accumulation of CSF due to imbalance between production and absorption of cerebrospinal fluid [126, 127]. The mechanism of dilatation of cerebral vessels is complex. Various factors play a significant role in different stages of its development.

The following factors are responsible for onset and progress of dilatation of the cerebral ventricles in hydrocephalus [5]:

1. Compression of vascular system, which can be compressed.

2. Redistribution of cerebrospinal fluid and extracellular fluid in CNS.

3. Changes of biomechanical properties of the brain (compliance of the brain tissue, disruption of viscoelastic properties of the brain).

4. Effect of pulse pressure of cerebrospinal fluid.

5. Loss of brain tissue accompanied by enlargement of the cerebral ventricles.

6. Increase of total volume of the skull resulting from effects of abnormal pressure on functional sutures in the skull of small children. In this age, additive cranial volume is the main factor of increase of volume of cerebrospinal fluid and enlargement of the cerebral ventricles [128].

Generally, in obstructive hydrocephalus, it is assumed that there is a significant pressure gradient between the cerebral ventricles, which is proximal to the site of obstruction of the CSF pathways and the subarachnoid space on convexity.

M. A. Williams et al.

TABLE 1

Research priorities for hydrocephalus

- *Hydrocephalus Research Infrastructure*
  - Creation of research networks
    - Basic, clinical, translational, & interdisciplinary research
  - Facilitation of information sharing
    - Specimen banks: brain, CSF, genetic material, shunts, images, physiological measurements
    - Registries: clinical trials, epidemiological data, longitudinal studies
  - Education & career development for researchers
    - Scientist & clinician/scientist education
- *Basic Research*
  - Injury & recovery mechanisms in human volunteers or animal models
    - Molecular, cellular, genetic, & systems physiology
      - Role of stem cells & neural progenitor cells
      - Role of inflammation, tissue matrix, blood–brain barrier, biomarkers
    - Anatomy & physiology of CSF secretion, circulation, resorption, function
    - Development of appropriate animal models for age, acuity of onset, & mode of induction factors, including congenital & acquired hydrocephalus
      - Ex vivo models (brain slices, tissue culture)
      - Transgenic models
  - Development & validation of theoretical & biomechanical modeling
    - CBF/CSF pulsatility, compartment models, ICP gradients, & monitoring
    - Physiological effects of CSF diversion, including slit-ventricle syndrome
- *Clinical Research*
  - Diagnosis
    - Establishment & validation of diagnostic criteria at all stages of life
    - Improvement & validation of imaging & noninvasive testing techniques
  - Current treatment, outcomes, complications
    - Epidemiology & population impact
    - Surgical treatment
      - Establishment & validation of treatment criteria at all stages of life
      - Prevention of infection & device or treatment failure
      - Effects of device design, biomaterials, & technique on outcomes
    - Clinical evaluation of brain/neuronal dysfunction & recovery
      - Development & validation of clinical conventions or templates for assessing neurological & behavioral outcomes (for example, cognitive, gait, motor, continence, activities of daily living)
      - Correlation of clinical outcomes w/ imaging & noninvasive techniques
      - Effects of infection & device or treatment failure on outcomes
    - Health services research
      - Education of patients, public, physician communities
      - Determination of extent of need for centers of excellence
      - Determination of extent of need for longitudinal care for children & adults w/ chronic hydrocephalus
      - Development of age-appropriate quality of life instruments
- *Future Treatments*
  - Development of adjunctive (pharmacological) therapies
  - Development of novel medical devices & biomaterials

Figure 16.
The list of priorities for hydrocephalus research. They were defined at the international congress National Institutes of Health (NIH)-sponsored workshop Hydrocephalus: Myths, New Facts, and Clear Directions held from September 29 to October 1, 2005, in Bethesda, Maryland (Williams et al., 2007).

However, the results of measurements confirmed that the pressure gradient is very low or zero. Even the low gradient between the cerebral ventricles and the subarachnoid space on convexity can cause onset and development of dilatation of the cerebral ventricles. The final value of intracranial pressure depends on transmission of the intraventricular pressure through the cerebral tissue toward the surface of the brain, which is influenced mainly by elastic properties of the brain tissue. If the brain tissue is less compressible (low compliance of the brain tissue), then transmission of pressure is significant, which leads to *tension hydrocephalus*. If the brain tissue is more compressible (higher compliance of the brain tissue), then transmission of pressure from the intraventricular compartment toward the brain surface is lower, which results in *normotensive hydrocephalus* [129]. The important role of viscoelastic properties of the brain and changes of CSF absorption in the development of the cerebral ventricle dilatation has been confirmed also by other researchers [130, 131].

Klarica et al. [132] performed the experiment with cats, which confirmed that obstruction of aqueduct is not the single cause of development of hypertensive acute hydrocephalus (induced by obstruction of aqueduct). Instillation of fluid into the cerebral ventricles, which are proximal to the site of obstruction, leads to development of pressure gradient between the cerebral ventricles and cisterna magna. After instillation of fluid, the pressure gradient diminished. However, pressure in the subarachnoid space, which acted on cerebrospinal fluid in the cerebral ventricles through the brain tissue, had increased during instillation of fluid into cisterna magna.

Peña et al. [133] also confirmed that in acute obstructive hydrocephalus, the degree of dilatation of cerebral ventricles depends on pressure gradient between the cerebral ventricles and the subarachnoid space. Development of periventricular edema was dependent on expansive (tension) forces acting on the brain tissue near the frontal and occipital horns of lateral cerebral ventricles. On the other hand, a concave shape of the lateral cerebral ventricle resulted in the development of compressive forces in the adjacent brain tissue. The results of the research confirmed that distribution of periventricular edema in acute hydrocephalus is independent on the intraventricular pressure as well as on geometrics of the cerebral ventricles.

Examination of cerebrospinal fluid by nuclear magnetic resonance showed that almost every movement of CSF is pulse in its nature. This provides evidence that hyperdynamic pulsations of the choroid plexus in communicating hydrocephalus are not only necessary but also sufficient for induction of dilatation of the cerebral ventricles. Communicating hydrocephalus can be developed also due to redistribution of CSF pulsations in the intracranial space [134].

Beside other factors, dilatation of cerebral ventricles also depends on the age of a child. Mechanic properties of the brain of a preterm neonate lead to preferential dilatation of posterior parts of lateral cerebral ventricles. This phenomenon can be defined by two mechanisms: increased compliance of the posterior part of the skull before cranial suture closure and decreased distensibility of the anterior part of the cerebral ventricles, which is surrounded by compact gray matter of the basal ganglia [5].

Increased production of cerebrospinal fluid is almost always present in tumors or villous hypertrophy of *plexus choroideus*, especially in papilloma or carcinoma of choroidal plexus [135, 136]. The increase of CSF production itself leads to increase of intracranial pressure and dilatation of the cerebral ventricles [137]. It must be emphasized that factors such as compression of CSF pathways, fibrosis of subarachnoid spaces, or villi arachnoidales due to microbleeding, which may increase

CSF flow resistance, occur in patients with tumor of the choroid plexus. Even though the patients underwent resection of tumor, increased production persists. Increased production of cerebrospinal fluid was confirmed also in hypervitaminosis A [5].

Obstruction of CSF pathways is a common cause of hydrocephalus. The obstruction can be either *intraventricular* (mainly in narrow inner CSF pathways) or *extraventricular* (obliteration of outer CSF pathways such as basal cisterns and subarachnoid spaces on convexity). Dilatation of cerebral ventricles depends on a site of obstruction. According to this, we can distinguish *hydrocephalus of one, two, three, or four ventricles*.

The obstruction of the CSF flow may develop due to various pathological conditions:

- Malformations, which lead to local constriction of CSF pathways (e.g., stenosis of *aqueductus (Sylvii)*)
- Expansive processes leading to compression of CSF pathways (tumors, arachnoid cysts, hematomas)
- Inflammatory processes—infections, fibrous changes after bleeding and inflammation, diseases (e.g., mucopolysaccharidosis), which induce ependymal reaction, leptomeningeal fibrosis, and obliteration of arachnoid villi

Increase of venous pressure in dural sinus results in two consequences:

1. Increase of venous pressure in the cerebral cortex leads to increase of intracranial venous volume.
2. Increase of intracranial pressure above the level, which is needed to ensure CSF flow in contrast to increase of venous pressure in the sinus.

Increase of venous pressure in the sinus may be of organic (thrombosis in the sinus, jugular vessels, or superior vena cava, spread of tumor to the sinus, achondroplasia) or functional (high-flow arteriovenous malformations) origin [18, 138].

6.2 Pathologic changes in hydrocephalus

Dilatation of the cerebral ventricles and increase of intracranial pressure in active hydrocephalus result in various pathological changes [139].

Ependyma of the cerebral ventricles is highly vulnerable. In the acute phase, ependymal cells are flattened, and ciliary apparatus is damaged. In the advanced phase, disruption of ependymal basal membrane can be seen. Eventually, the ependymal membrane is seriously damaged, and the surface of cerebral ventricles is covered by glial tissue. Ependymal cells have atypical surface. They are distorted, and desmosomes are damaged [140]. Nakamura and Sato [141] emphasized that ciliary dyskinesis in *aqueductus (Sylvii)* might be one of the factors, which have impact on the development of hydrocephalus.

The cortical mantle is diminished and stretched due to dilatation of cerebral ventricles and increased intracranial pressure. Character and distribution of pathological changes depend on age, in which hydrocephalus has developed, development rate, size of cerebral ventricle dilatation, and duration of hydrocephalus. In the acute phase, edema of periventricular white matter is present. And neurons are not damaged too much. In the advanced stage, edema of white matter diminished and is substituted by fibrotic changes and axon degeneration (demyelination), which is responsible for brain atrophy and focal decrease of neurons [142, 143]. Brain damage results from the combination of mechanic distortion and cerebral blood flow disorder (distortion of cerebral vessels, compression of cerebral capillaries). Cortical dysgenesis may occur in the early onset of dilatation of cerebral ventricles [144].

Changes in cerebral cortex after drainage procedure include major regeneration of myelin of residual axons and astroglial proliferation with mesenchymal reaction, especially in capillaries. Increase of neuron fibers was not confirmed. The extent of damage of the cerebral cortex is a critical moment for regeneration of cortical mantle in chronic hydrocephalus [145]. Drainage procedure provides only partial regeneration of the brain tissue. Damage of dendrites persists. This has negative impact on the development of connections between neurons during postsurgical recovery [144, 146].

Among other pathological changes in the development of hydrocephalus, there are perforations of septum pellucidum, ventrolateral compression of nucleus caudatus, and compression of cerebellum hemispheres with erosion on their surface [147].

Azzi et al. [148] emphasize causal relationship between increased intracranial pressure, dilatation of cerebral ventricles, and cerebral edema, which is responsible for hydrocephalus. Alteration of the parameters occurs rather in sequences than simultaneously, and the course of manifestations of hydrocephalus is different.

The difference between total volume of free water and bound water, which is contained in the cerebral cortex, was not found in any stage of hydrocephalus. Any evidence of change was found in total volume of water in periventricular white matter. But in acute and subacute stages of hydrocephalus, total volume of free water was increased, while volume of bound water was decreased. In the chronic stage, values of free and bound water were in standard range. In acute and subacute stages of hydrocephalus, free water flows through ependymal lining of cerebral ventricles into the periventricular white matter, which results in decrease of volume of free water. In chronic hydrocephalus, employment of alternative drainage pathways enables drainage of free water from the periventricular white matter, so volume of free water is back in standard values [149]. When volume of free water in the periventricular white matter is increased, alteration of energetic metabolism is present. Employment of alternative drainage pathways decreases edema of the white matter and improves energetic state of the white matter of the brain [150].

Increase of intracranial pressure in pediatric hydrocephalus may cause *disorders of the autonomous nervous system and regulation of body temperature* [151]. When it is accompanied by dysfunction of the autonomous nervous system, then dysfunction of cerebral cortex, subcortical structures, and cerebral stem develops. When drainage procedure was performed in neonates with active hydrocephalus, dysfunction of cardiac regulation has improved [152, 153].

6.3 Vascular changes in hydrocephalus

Changes in nerve tissue are accompanied by alteration of the vascular system, which may improve if hydrocephalus is treated early and appropriately [5]. Distortion of cerebral vessels, compression and collapse of capillaries, and disorder of cerebral circulation occur. The vascular system of periventricular white matter and cerebral cortex is usually most damaged. Damage of the cerebral system involves development and worsening of ischemic damage and alteration of energetic cerebral metabolism (**Figure 17**).

The degree and type of changes of cerebral circulation depend on the development and course of hydrocephalus. Compression of capillaries, also called

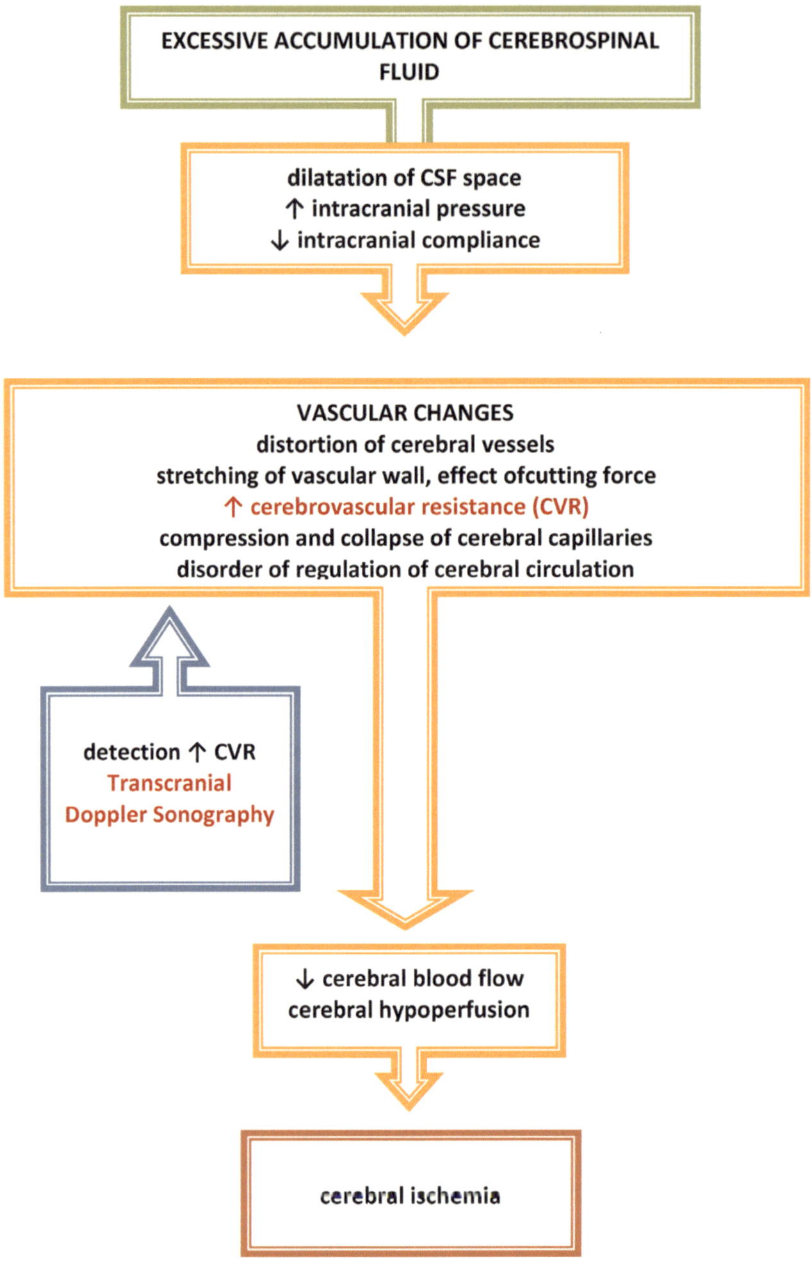

Figure 17.
The flowchart diagram of changes of cerebral circulation during development of progressive hydrocephalus.

cerebrovascular compression, plays a significant role in the *acute stage*. Various research studies have confirmed collapse of cerebral capillaries in the periventricular white matter and cortical and subcortical gray matter [154–158]. Changes of cerebral circulation, which are adaptive in their nature, also known as cerebrovascular adaptation, occur in the *chronic stage* of hydrocephalus. Their role is to ensure appropriate cerebral perfusion and metabolic demands of the brain. Development and employment of adaptive processes require time, so they are preferred mainly in slowly progressive hydrocephalus.

In the experimental study with dogs, Luciano et al. [159] confirmed that adaptive changes of cerebral circulation appeared 10–12 weeks after induction of hydrocephalus. After initial decrease of vascular supply of the cerebral tissue (collapse of cerebral capillaries), they found out that cerebral circulation in the periventricular white matter, nucleus caudatus, and cerebral cortex can be restored in chronic hydrocephalus. An increased number of cerebral capillaries, confirmed by histological examination, may be caused by continuous blood flow in capillaries as well as capillary angiogenesis in chronic hypoxic condition.

In chronic hydrocephalus, the protective effect of nimodipine has been proven in experimental studies. It improved blood flow in periventricular white matter but did not affect proteolytic processes in axons due to Ca^{2+} influx [160].

da Silva et al. [161] observed changes of cerebral blood flow in cats with kaolin-induced hydrocephalus. They found out that ICBF in the cerebral cortex, white matter, and subcortical structures of the gray matter was decreased 1 week after hydrocephalus induction.

The biggest decrease of ICBF was confirmed in the white matter of the parietal lobe. Three weeks after hydrocephalus induction, decrease of ICBF persisted only in the white matter (in the parietal lobe, occipital lobe, and corpus callosum), while perfusion of cerebral cortex and deep subcortical structures had returned to normal values.

Observation of changes of cerebral perfusion and metabolism has brought new knowledge also about pathophysiology of normotensive hydrocephalus [162–164].

6.4 Biochemical changes in hydrocephalus

Studies on potential *prognostic markers of brain damage in hydrocephalus* have shown an increased amount of proteins in cerebrospinal fluid and change of electrophoretic spectrum of proteins in various conditions of hydrocephalus [165]. Concentration of fatty acids, xanthine, hypoxanthine, ganglioside GM1, and lactate in cerebrospinal fluid seems to be an interesting prognostic factor [166–169].

A role of neuronal death in pathophysiology is not clear. Ding et al. [170] found out that neuronal death did not play a main role in experimental hydrocephalus. However, when acute ischemia was induced in the frontal lobe of the brain in rats with hydrocephalus, increased tolerance of neurons to ischemia has been confirmed.

Shinoda et al. [171] proved increased *expression of neurotrophins and their receptors* in damaged structures of the brain in rats.

Experiments have shown that besides other mechanisms, also *Ca^{2+}-activated proteolytic processes* cause damage of periventricular white matter in hydrocephalus [172].

Caner et al. [173] in their study revealed an increased level of lipid peroxidation of the cerebral vessels. It might be a result of ischemia caused by stretching of cerebral vessels in hydrocephalus.

Onset and development of hydrocephalus leads to alteration of *neurotransmitter systems* in the brain. Tashiro et al. [174] confirmed that mechanic distortion in progressive hydrocephalus causes functional damage of cholinergic and GABAergic neurons in neostriatum and dopaminergic neurons in the substantia nigra compacta. Disorders of neurotransmitter signals in the basal ganglia may explain some of the functional motoric disorders in hydrocephalus. Chovanes et al. [175] found out that the level of noradrenaline (71%), dopamine (73%), and serotonin (50%) was decreased in the cerebral cortex, neostriatum, and cerebellum. The level of noradrenaline and serotonin was increased in the brain stem. This might be a sign of axonal transport deficit from the locus ceruleus to the raphe area.

Hydrocephalus is associated with progressive malfunction and destruction of axons and neurons. Growth-associated protein 43 is responsible for neuroaxonal regeneration and synaptic remodelation. In the early stage of hydrocephalus, the level of growth-associated protein 43 increases in periventricular axons.

This shows how important early intervention in prevention and restoration of axonal damage in hydrocephalus is. Increased expression of growth-associated protein 43 in the cerebral cortex is a sign of alteration of cortical synaptogenesis [176]. Suda et al. [177] observed the level of synaptic vesicle-associated protein 38 (SVP-38) and developmentally regulated brain proteins (drebrins) in rats with congenital hydrocephalus. Their study confirmed alteration of synaptogenesis in prenatal period, which had been restored after early drainage procedure.

The glutamate/aspartate transporter (GLAST) system plays a significant role in maintaining the extracellular concentration of glutamate below neurotoxic level. Masago et al. [178] confirmed GLAST expression in the reactive astrocytes in the periventricular white matter and regulation of glutamate concentration in hydrocephalus.

Increased concentration of *vascular endothelial growth factor* (VEGF) *and erythropoietin* (*EPO*) in cerebrospinal fluid was confirmed in neonates and children with active hydrocephalus. The levels increased due to brain tissue hypoxia, which stimulates expression of genes for EPO and VEGF [179].

6.5 Changes of cerebral metabolism in hydrocephalus

Changes of energetic and membrane metabolism of the brain tissue play a significant role in pathogenesis of hydrocephalus. The changes can be described in detail by in vitro and in vivo nuclear magnetic spectroscopy.

Tamaki et al. [180] performed an experiment using in vivo 31P-MR spectroscopy. The experiment revealed decreased the ratio between organic creatine phosphate and inorganic phosphate, which is an indicator of bioenergetic state (energetic index) in acute and subacute stages of hydrocephalus. Restoration of the ratio between organic creatine phosphate and inorganic phosphate was found in the chronic stage of hydrocephalus. Decrease of adenosine triphosphate was not confirmed in any of these stages.

da Silva et al. [181] observed changes of energetic metabolism in hydrocephalus and impact of drainage procedure (VP shunt insertion) on energetic condition of the brain tissue. The experiment revealed decrease of the ratio between organic creatine phosphate and inorganic phosphate and increase of the ratio between inorganic phosphate and ATP. Direct correlation between energetic index and size of cerebral ventricles was confirmed. When drainage procedure was performed, periventricular edema diminished, cerebral ventricles decreased, and the ratio of organic creatine phosphate/inorganic phosphate and the ratio of inorganic phosphate/ATP return to normal values. The results show that hypoxic-ischemic encephalopathy accompanied by malfunction of energetic metabolism, which can be reversible if drainage procedure is performed early, occurs in active hydrocephalus.

Braun et al. [182] used 1H MR spectroscopy to observe changes in the brain tissue in adult rats. Malfunction and structural damage of neurons and membrane systems can be detected when the level of neurometabolites is examined. The results showed increase of lactate and decrease of pH. Moreover, decrease of ratio N-acetylaspartate/choline and ratio of creatine/choline was found out in the acute as well as chronic stage of hydrocephalus. This is a sign of neural dysfunction, neural destruction, changes of phospholipid metabolism in membranes, and myelin damage.

Harris et al. [183] observed changes of neurometabolites in the cerebral cortex. The experiment showed decrease of myoinositol, creatine, choline, N-acetylaspartate, taurine, glutamine, glutamate, aspartate, alanine, glycine, GABA, and phosphocreatine.

7. Clinical manifestations of pediatric hydrocephalus

Signs of dilatation of the frontal horns of lateral cerebral ventricles (apathy) and dilatation of aqueduct and the third cerebral ventricle (oculomotor dysfunction) and signs of intracranial hypertension are clinical manifestations of active hydrocephalus in children. *Clinical signs of intracranial hypertension* can be divided into *anatomic* (the biomechanical properties of calva—diastasis of cerebral sutures, enlarged and bulged fontanelles, bigger size of the head) and *signs associated with the homeostasis of intracranial space* such as vomiting, quantitative disturbance of consciousness, breathing pattern disorders, bradycardia, and oculomotor dysfunction [184, 185]. Other clinical manifestations of pediatric hydrocephalus are noticeable and enlarged veins of calva caused by reverse blood flow from cerebral veins due to increased intracranial pressure and a cracked pot sign.

Manifestation of clinical signs of intracranial hypertension depends on course of hydrocephalus, age of a child, fibroelastic and biomechanical properties of the cranium, and employment of compensation mechanisms. Clinical signs of intracranial hypertension vary widely mainly in babies (neonates and infants). After cerebral suture closure and ossification of the calva, the skull gets biomechanical properties of the skulls of an adult. This is the cause of uniform clinical manifestation of increased intracranial pressure in older child age categories. In older children, hydrocephalus may manifest with headache, worse school results, or changes in behavior [186, 187].

According to course of hydrocephalus, we can distinguish acute hydrocephalus with need of immediate drainage procedure, progressive hydrocephalus, and chronic compensated hydrocephalus either with subcompensation of intermittent episodes or immediate decompensation. Severe decompensation of hydrocephalus with rapid deterioration of neurological condition is rare in children (unconsciousness, low values at Glasgow coma scale, development of bilateral mydriasis accompanied by defects of photoreaction, breathing pattern disorders, bradycardia). If the anterior fontanelle is not closed, puncture of the lateral cerebral ventricle through the anterior fontanelle is immediately performed. It is an urgent procedure performed during cerebral resuscitation. The Chiraflex needle can be used for the urgent puncture of the lateral cerebral ventricle. It can be combined with intravenous cannula, which helps to measure intracranial pressure. Then cerebrospinal fluid derivation is done by aspiration. The amount of derived CSF depends on an individual (age of a child, CSF production, size of CSF pathways). The amount of aspired cerebrospinal fluid should decrease ICP to the values of 10–12 cm H_2O. This will lead to temporary compensation of the condition, in which detailed diagnosis (if it was not done before the ventricular puncture due to lack of time) and immediate surgery can be performed. If the anterior fontanelle is closed, trepanation is performed in the frontal part of the skull at the right side with insertion of external ventricular drainage. If cerebrospinal fluid derivation is not done quickly and effectively in a child with severe decompensated hydrocephalus, there is only a low chance for a good neurological effect of the drainage procedure [188].

Some signs of intracranial hypertension (apathy, somnolence, vomiting, irritability, and breathing pattern disorders) are *nonspecific* and may occur also in other illnesses. Usually they occur in infections of the upper and lower airways, gastroenteritis, or in infection of the uropoetic system. They may imitate activity of hydrocephalus or failure of the internal drainage system, especially in neonates and young children with hydrocephalus. On the other hand, infection, which occurs in compensated hydrocephalus without need of drainage, may lead to decompensation of the stationary state, in which a drainage procedure is necessary [189].

In active hydrocephalus, the head size of neonates and infants increases due to diastasis of cranial sutures and fontanelles (**Figures 18–23**). There is high variability of biomechanical properties of the skull in a particular age group; therefore, manifestation of the signs will be different. It is important to take measures of three dimensions: circumference of the head, lateral and ventrodorsal. While a child is staying in hospital, the same nurse should measure his head. Then the measures are being compared with the referential values in relation to the gestation age of a child. The percentile graph with assessment scale of head circumference is usually used in

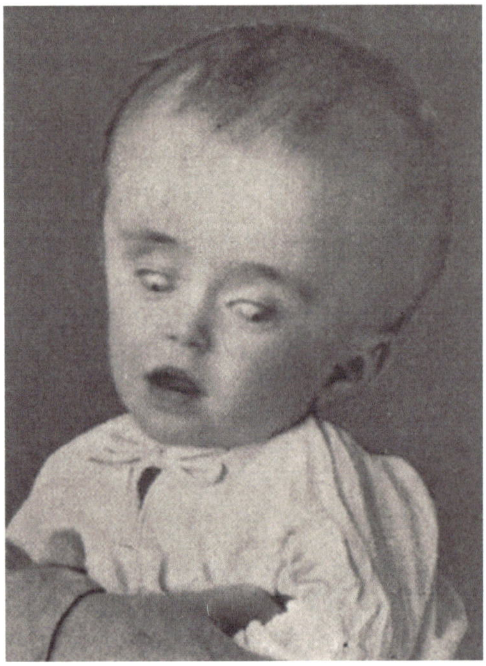

Figure 18.
A child with hydrocephalus. The enlarged head and sunset eye sign. Source: [21].

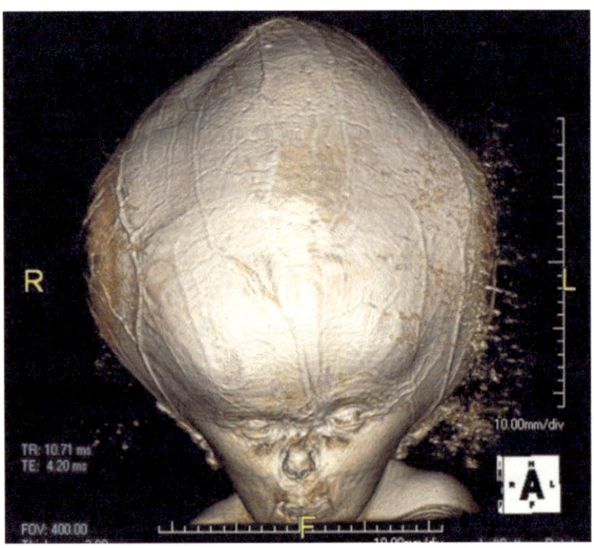

Figure 19.
Three-dimensional reconstruction of the CT image of child's head with hydrocephalus.

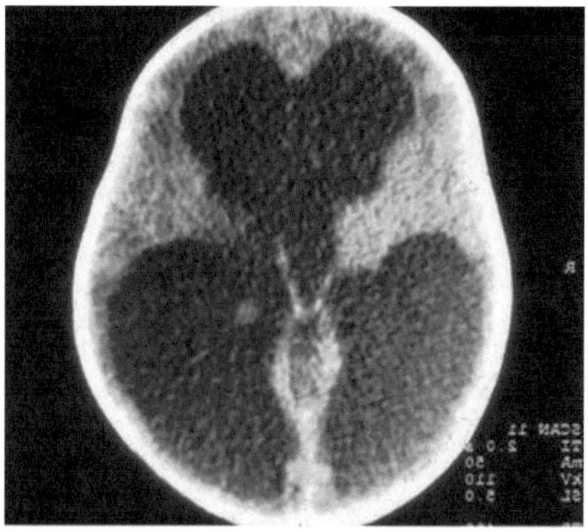

Figure 20.
CT image of hydrocephalus. Distinct dilatation of the cerebral ventricles and periventricular hypodensity are apparent.

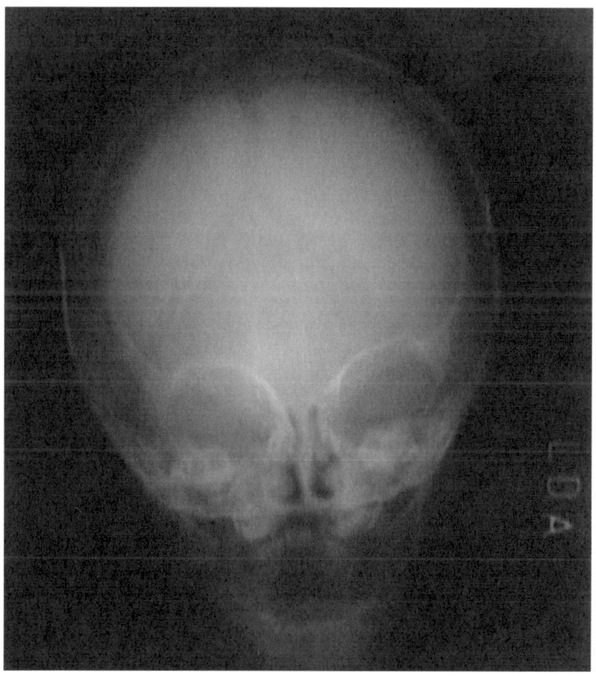

Figure 21.
X-ray image of the child's head with active hydrocephalus. Enlarged head, apparent diastasis of the sagittal and lambdoid sutures.

clinical practice (**Figure 24**) [190]. Before a child is discharged from a hospital, his parents are informed about clinical manifestations of increased intracranial pressure and drainage system failure and how to measure head circumference. Parents should be given the child's identity card, which contains information about insertion of the drainage system and contact details of the department where the shunt procedure was performed. After discharge, the parents should measure the circumference of child's head at least once a week and take records of the measures [186, 191].

The diastasis of sagittal and lambdoid suture is examined by palpation of a child's head. Enlargement of the lambdoid suture is considered pathognomonic. Enlargement of the cranial sutures can be seen at X-ray or CT scan of the skull

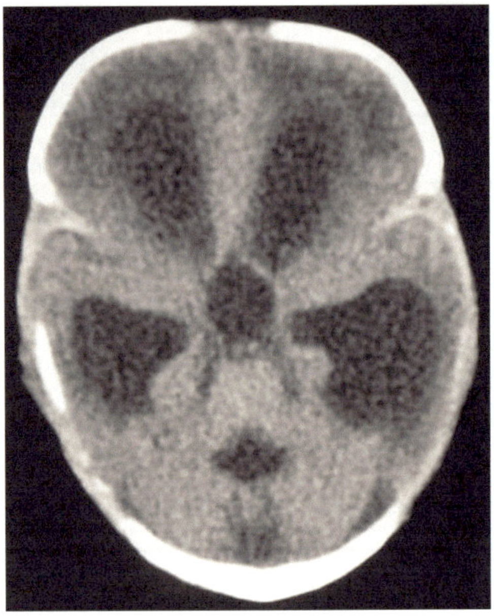

Figure 22.
CT image of the infant's brain with active hydrocephalus. Apparent dilatation of the cerebral ventricles, diastasis of cranial sutures, and periventricular hypodensities.

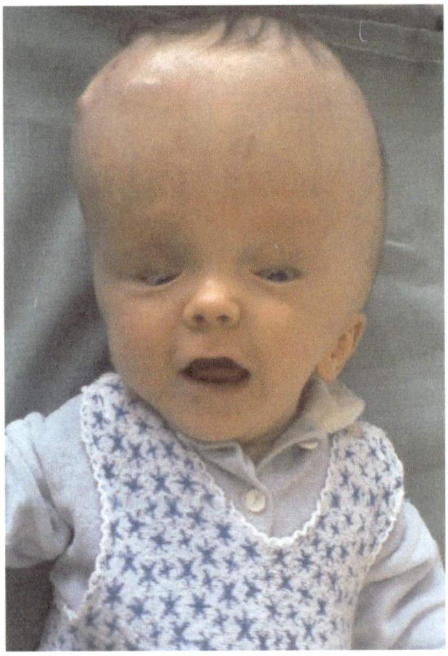

Figure 23.
A child with hydrocephalus with a ventriculoperitoneal shunt.

(**Figures 21** and **22**). *The anterior fontanelle is usually bulged over niveau, enlarged and hard when palpated*. However, palpation examination of the anterior fontanelle might be ambiguous even though the intracranial pressure is increased. If compliance of the brain tissue is increased (in hypoxic-ischemic encephalopathy, in inflammatory processes in the brain), the cerebral ventricles may enlarge significantly during the initial stage of increase of intracranial pressure, and clinical manifestations of intracranial hypertension don't have to be manifested clearly, without any change in the anterior fontanelle and cranial sutures. On the contrary,

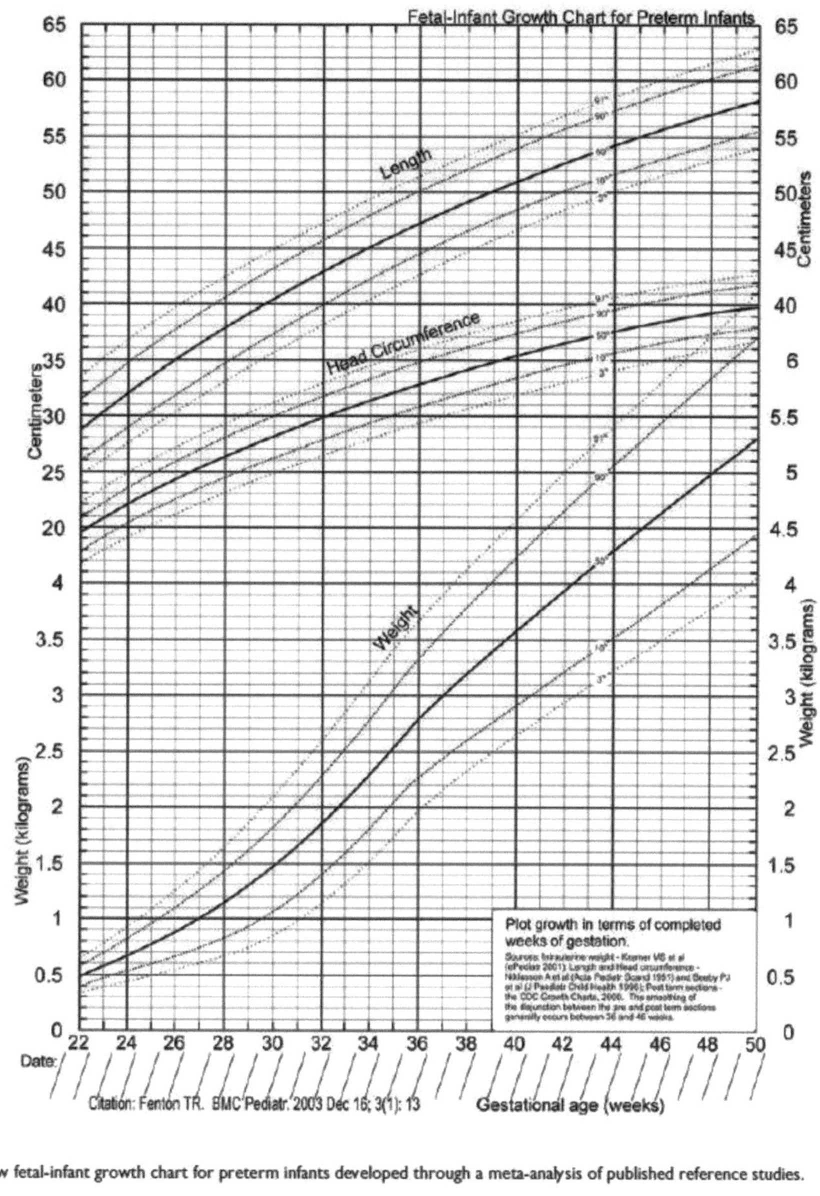

Figure 24.
The percentile graph with findings of head circumference, length of the body, and weight in preterm neonates [190].

hypoxic-ischemic encephalopathy or brain damage caused by inflammation may result in reduction of cerebral tissue and hydrocephalus ex vacuo without increase of intracranial pressure [189].

Variability of clinical manifestations of intracranial hypertension, especially in young children, may be a complication for indication of drainage procedure in children with hydrocephalus. Despite the dysfunction of cerebrospinal fluid dynamics and increased intracranial pressure, the clinical signs of intracranial hypertension might be manifested only partially or not at all [192–194].

For this reason, in assessment of pediatric hydrocephalus, we have also focused on the analysis of clinical signs of intracranial hypertension in neonates and infants. The statistical methods were used to describe significance of chosen clinical signs, which are linked to urgent indication of drainage procedure. The results showed that the drainage procedure was indicated early and appropriately, without waiting for further progression in the clinical findings of a child. The clinical signs, which have the highest sensitivity in relation to indication of the drainage procedure, in neonates and infants with hydrocephalus, are increased head circumference (72%), progression of head circumference (61%), tense anterior fontanelle in palpation (56%), and diastasis of cranial sutures (56%). The clinical signs of intracranial hypertension with the highest specificity are bulged anterior fontanelle (99%), progression of head circumference (98%), tense anterior fontanelle in palpation (91%), and diastasis of lambdoid suture (88%). The most positive value of the Youden index was found in progression of head circumference. The value of the Youden index for nonspecific signs of intracranial hypertension (apathy, somnolence, vomiting, sundown syndrome, and irritability) was very low (**Table 4**) [195].

Besides common clinical signs, less common or rare manifestations, such as torticollis, opisthotonus, dilatation of vessels in the face, episodes of whistling and screaming, hothead syndrome, occur in children with hydrocephalus [196]. In some cases, hydrocephalus may manifest with spasms and epileptic seizures. Especially in preterm neonates with posthemorrhagic or postinfectious hydrocephalus, subclinical seizures may be detected bedside by aEEG (**Figure 25**).

The results of the studies confirmed that clinical signs might not show the real value of intracranial pressure [197–199]. Indirect measuring of ICP by a tonometer or Ladd ICP monitor, which can be used to examine ICP values, is limited by a wide range of findings and high subjectivity of examination [28].

Clinical signs	Sensitivity (%)	Specificity (%)	False-positive result (%)	False-negative result (%)	Youden index
Diastasis of cranial sutures	56	65	35	45	0.205
Diastasis of sagittal suture	56	65	35	45	0.205
Diastasis of lambdoid suture	42	**88**	12	58	0.297
Bulged fontanelle	**31**	**99**	1	69	0.296
Tense fontanelle in palpation	**56**	**91**	9	44	**0.461**
Soft fontanelle	14	15	85	86	−**0.713**
Increased head circumference	**72**	72	28	28	0.44
Progression of head Circumference	**61**	**98**	2	39	**0.593**
Sundown syndrome	8	95	5	92	0.033
Vomiting	14	92	8	86	0.062
Breathing pattern disorders	0	92	8	100	−0.077
Apathy, somnolence	33	86	14	67	0.196
Irritability	11	80	20	89	−0.094

The significance for bold values is $p \leq 0,05$.

Table 4.
Assessment of clinical signs of intracranial hypertension in relation to indication of drainage procedure in neonates and infants with hydrocephalus [195].

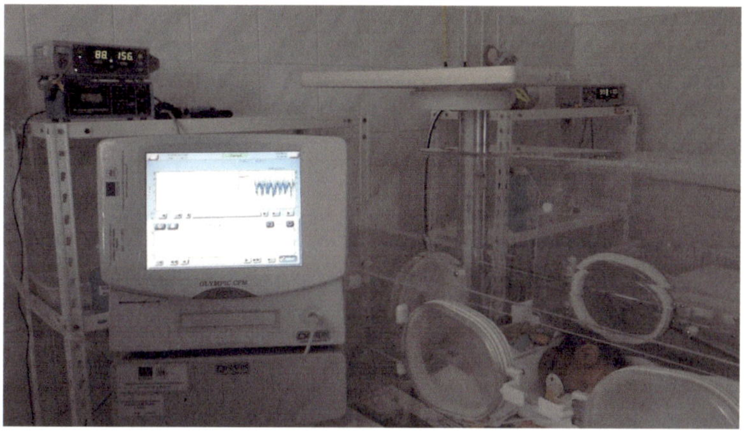

Figure 25.
Monitoring of epileptic activity in the preterm neonate with intraventricular hemorrhage by aEEG.

Direct measurement of intracranial pressure is not routinely performed when assessing indication of the drainage procedure, because it is invasive and may cause complications in children with hydrocephalus. If diagnosis is not clear and clinical symptomatology indicates dysfunction of cerebrospinal fluid dynamics and increased intracranial pressure, invasive methods, for example, ICP screening followed by ICP monitoring and infusion tests, are being used [196]. In neonates and infants with hydrocephalus, ICP value is usually measured during ventricular or lumbar puncture, which was performed to take a sample of cerebrospinal fluid for biochemical and microbiological examination. The value of intracranial pressure may be measured during surgery, which will confirm intracranial hypertension and appropriate indication of drainage procedure. Moreover, a neurosurgeon may use the intraoperative ICP values to setting the opening pressure in programmable valves of the drainage system (**Figure 26**).

Regarding various measurement methods, normal and abnormal ICP values will differ among neonates with low birth weight. For noninvasive methods of ICP measurement, which employ optic fibers [200] and pneumatic-tonometric sensors [201],

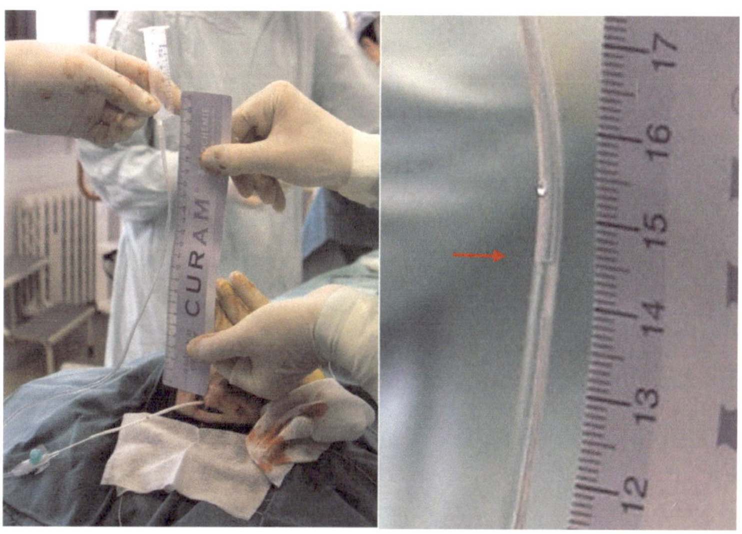

Figure 26.
Direct measurement of intracranial pressure during insertion of VP shunt in the neonate with hydrocephalus (ICP +14.5 cm in column of CSF).

the normal value in healthy neonates ranges from 4.5 to 7.0 cm H_2O. The normal values of ICP measured during lumbar puncture range from 3 to 7 cm H_2O [28]. The accurate value, which determines development of progressive dilatation of the cerebral ventricles in neonates, is not clear. Generally, the ICP value must be higher than the normal ICP value. Regarding high volume of water, low level of myelin, increase in cerebral compliance, and enlarged subarachnoid space of the brain in preterm neonates, the ICP value, which determines onset and development of progressive dilatation of cerebral ventricles, might be lower [28, 202]. Generally, in lying children, the normal ICP value is 12 ± 2 cm H_2O. In neonates and infants, the normal values of intracranial pressure are lower (ICP ≤ 6 cm H_2O for preterm neonates and ICP ≤ 10 cm H_2O for term neonates and infants).

The use of *drainage systems (shunts)* plays an important role in the treatment of pediatric hydrocephalus (**Figure 27**). In the survey of 1791 patients, up to 56% of them had experienced at least one episode of dysfunction of the drainage system during 12 years since the shunt had been inserted [203]. Similarly, Lazareff et al. [204] confirmed that 44% out of 224 children had experienced a dysfunction of the drainage system during 6 years since the shunt had been inserted. The highest risk of dysfunction is in the first year of a shunt insertion. Some authors observed malfunction of VP shunt in the first year of insertion in 40% of cases [205–207]. The overview of the most common complications of the drainage systems is shown in **Table 5**.

Regarding a high risk of complications associated with the drainage systems [208, 209], the endoscopic surgery is currently preferred in pediatric hydrocephalus [210]. Endoscopic procedures in children with hydrocephalus usually include ventriculostomy of the third cerebral ventricle (**Figure 28**), aqueductoplasty, septoplasty, and removal of the intraventricular tumors and cysts [211]. The results of various studies show that ETV is successful in 49–100% cases [212–219]. Increased risk of ETV failure has been found in posthemorrhagic and postinfectious hydrocephalus in infants under 1 year of age [220–222]. According to some authors [223], success of ETV is determined rather by etiology of hydrocephalus than by age of the child.

The value of intracranial pressure is often used in children with active hydrocephalus as an indicator of dysfunction of the ventriculoperitoneal shunt [224, 225]. Gilkes et al. [226] dealt with changes of the intracranial pressure and cerebral perfusion pressure in shunt-dependent children with hydrocephalus with VP shunt dysfunction

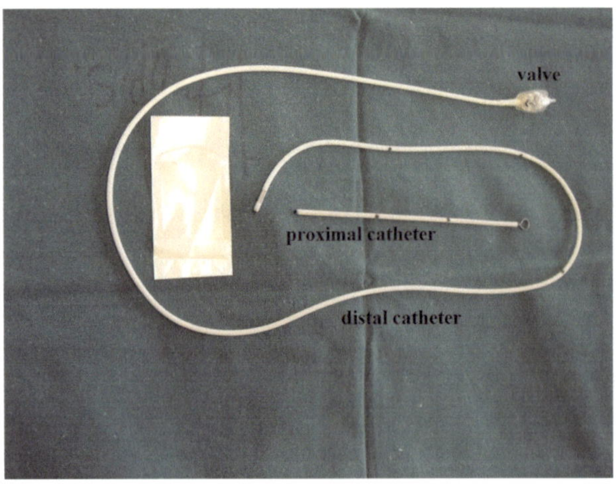

Figure 27.
The internal drainage system.

Noninfectious complications	Hyperdrainage condition	Slit ventricles syndrome, subdural collections
	Proximal part of drainage system	Dislocation and obstruction of ventricular catheter, subcutaneous CSF collection, CSF fistula and leak, wound dehiscence
	Valve	Dysfunction of valve, obstruction of valve, change of permeability in programmed valves, decubitus above valve, breakdown of the system
	Distal part of drainage system	Obstruction and dislocation of a distal catheter; VP shunt, migration of a catheter into the peritoneal cavity; CSF pseudocyst; VA shunt, migration of a catheter into the right cavities of the heart; thrombus; embolism in pulmonary artery; shunt nephritis; lung hypertension
Infectious complications (shunt infections)	Local infection in the wound and along the drainage system, ventriculitis, meningitis, meningoencephalitis, endocarditis, septicemia, lung abscesses, peritonitis	

Table 5.
The overview of the most common complications of drainage systems in pediatric hydrocephalus [208].

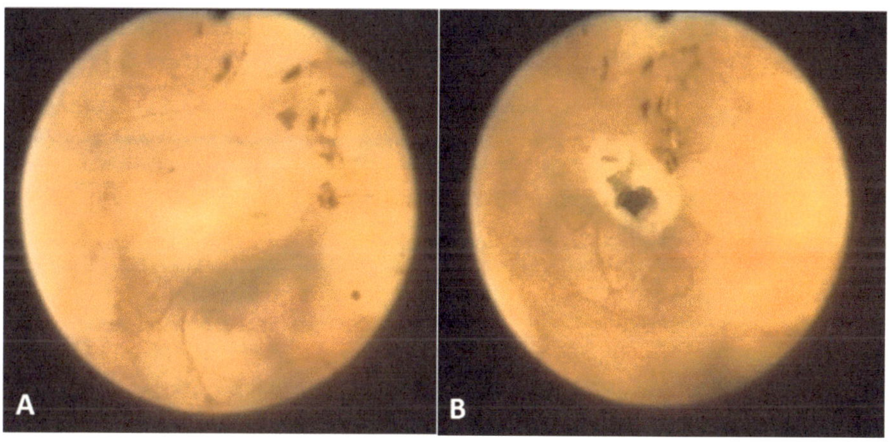

Figure 28.
Endoscopic view on the base of the third cerebral ventricle in the infant with a posthemorrhagic hydrocephalus with neuroinfection. Hemosiderin deposits are present, (A) before ETV, (B) after ETV.

linked to employment of compensation mechanisms. They found out that ICP was significantly lower in cases with the use of compensation mechanism than cases in which the compensation mechanisms were not employed at all. Even though ICP value is normal, dysfunction of the drainage system may be present anyway. The insufficient use of compensation mechanisms leads to ICP increase. When compensation mechanisms have been employed, the level of cerebral perfusion pressure was normal in 60% of cases compared to 30% if they have not been used.

In most cases dysfunction of drainage system in shunt-dependent children with hydrocephalus manifests with clinical signs of intracranial hypertension [227, 228]. Clinical manifestation of acute blockage of the drainage system is heterogeneous. High morbidity and mortality are common if it is not diagnosed and treated early. Clinical signs of intracranial hypertension might be very low or none. The common signs of dysfunction of drainage system are headache, vomiting, and drowsiness. The atypical signs are seizures, abdominal pseudocyst, syringomyelia, neural dysfunction, and hemiparesis [229]. Rigidity, visual impairment, and delay of psychomotor development of a child may occur as well.

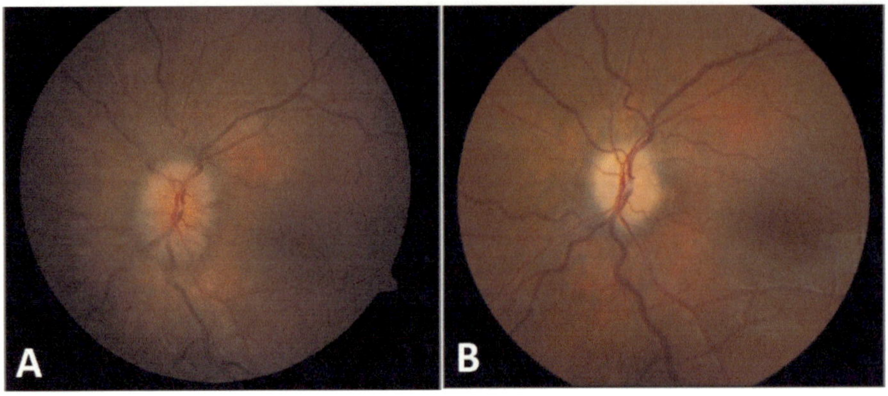

Figure 29.
Ophthalmological examination. (A) Edema of the optic nerve disc before a drainage procedure in hydrocephalus. (B) Correction by insertion of a shunt. Source: [236].

Presence of disease, which may manifest with similar clinical symptoms, e.g., respiratory infection, virosis, gastroenteritis, and infection of the uropoetic system, must be taken into consideration during examination of a child with hydrocephalus if dysfunction of the drainage system is suspected.

Regarding the age of a child and the fact that 60% of children with hydrocephalus attend special schools, lack of information in medical history provided by a child often causes problems in examination [120, 230, 231].

According to Barnes et al. [232], if headache, vomiting, and drowsiness occur together in a child with hydrocephalus who has the drainage system, there is a high risk of drainage system dysfunction, mostly acute blockage. Less common is shunt infection, especially in children without manifestation of increased body temperature. Strong positive correlation between drowsiness and acute blockage of drainage system has been found in statistical analysis of the clinical signs linked to drainage system dysfunction. There is weak predictive value of isolated headache or vomiting related to acute blockage drainage system. Therefore a child should be examined for the presence of other diseases. According to some authors [229, 233], the range of clinical signs in children with hydrocephalus with drainage system dysfunction (including infection) is as follows: headache (47–55%), vomiting (40–90%), and drowsiness (30–60%).

Arnell et al. [234] emphasize *the role of ophthalmologic examination* in drainage system dysfunction in shunt-dependent children with hydrocephalus. Loss of vision due to increased intracranial pressure and drainage system dysfunction has been described in literature, but the occurrence is not clear [235]. Loss of vision may be caused either by damage of the anterior optic tract, especially edema of the optic disc (**Figure 29**), atrophy of the optic disc, and slowed or missing reaction to light exposure, or by damage of the posterior optic tract resulting in cortical blindness [237–239]. In young children with hydrocephalus, increased intracranial pressure may occur independently on the presence of the optic disc edema [239, 240]. However, in older children, a regular ophthalmologic examination focused on the optic disc is recommended. This may help early detection of dysfunction of drainage system with some or only discretely manifested clinical signs of intracranial hypertension as well as in cases when CT image is not clear enough [234].

The parents play a significant role in clinical examination of a child. The parent's experience with episode of drainage system dysfunction must be taken into consideration when examining the child with hydrocephalus. A neurosurgeon examines the child once a year, or even less, if he relies on a general pediatrician. The parents know the child's daily routines the best so they can assess changes in his behavior.

Therefore, close cooperation between a doctor and the parents is a basic requirement for early detection of drainage system dysfunction [241].

8. Basic properties of ultrasound

Definition of ultrasound. The ultrasound waves are mechanical-elastic oscillations, which move in the matter. Their movement is enabled by elasticity and compactness of the matter. The frequency of oscillation of ultrasound is above the upper level, i.e., 20,000 Hz. The frequency of 2–10 MHz is used in medicine [242].

The ultrasound is a mechanic oscillation, which transits the area of hard particles and makes vibrations. Properties of vibrations depend on density and structure of the tissue. Instead of movement of the matter, energy spreads around. This kind of oscillation is called longitudinal [243]. Other types of oscillation (transversal, etc.) cannot spread around in the environment sufficiently.

The basic properties of the ultrasound are:

Frequency is measured in hertz (Hz) or in cycles per second.

Wavelength is a distance between compression of the same place of a medium in two successive cycles; it is measured in meters or corresponding subunits.

Movement velocity is determined by properties of environment, in which oscillation spreads around.

Pressure of waves depends on pressure oscillations related to counteractive static pressure (atmospheric, tissue).

Oscillation intensity is the spread of energy described by a unit of surface in a unit of time; it is measured in W/cm^2.

When applying ultrasound to the human body, two limitations need to be taken into consideration—distinguishing property and absorption of ultrasound in tissues. The shorter the wave distance is, the better the distinguishing property of an ultrasound is. But at the same time, ultrasound is more absorbed in tissues [242]. The human tissue is not a homogenous environment for spread of oscillation, so the oscillation is modified in various ways. It can be reflected off, refracted, broken apart, or absorbed.

If an ultrasound beam crosses the boundary of two environments, one part of the beam goes through it, while the other part reflects off. If the beam reflects off, the angle of reflection depends on the angle of incidence and acoustic impedance of two different environments. If the acoustic resistance of boundary environments differs significantly (e.g., tissue and gas), all energy can be reflected. Oscillation, which has not been reflected, subordinates to scattering. Then it interferes and part of it goes back through the boundary of the environments. This part may play a crucial role in the final interpretation of a sonographic image. The ability of the tissue to reflect echoes is called *echogenicity* (or *echogeneity*). The strongest reflections (echogenous and hyperechogenous) make large surfaces with high amount of collagen (the diaphragm, vessels, and sacs of the organs). The small surfaces containing low amount of collagen, which reflect narrow beams, are called hypoechogenous (parenchymal organs) [242].

9. Biological effects of ultrasound

Biological effects of ultrasound include all processes in the living tissue, which are caused by oscillation. It may induce them directly, or it serves as a trigger and facilitator factor for their onset and development [41].

Assessment of the ultrasound-induced biological effects and safety of ultrasound diagnostic method has become more complex because of advances in research and capacity regulation of the equipment. The modern sonographic equipment is more effective in diagnostic processes, but it produces higher acoustic intensity than the simple B-mode device [244].

Ultrasound examination is an inevitable part of diagnostic methods applied in neurological disorders not only in neonates and infants but also in adults. However, an increase of number and duration of examinations leads to higher exposure of the brain tissue to ultrasound oscillations. The harmful biological effects on patients and healthcare professionals exposed to ultrasound within the diagnostic power range have not been confirmed yet. However, types of damage caused by mechanisms, which have been already recognized, or by the new ones must be taken into consideration. The harmful effects of ultrasound examinations are still a disputed topic in literature [41].

The biological effect depends on properties of ultrasound oscillation and environment. Ultrasound is a mechanical form of energy, in which pressure wave goes through the tissue. In general, physical effects of ultrasound are classified as follows:

Thermal effects—overheating of the tissue after ultrasound transition; heat is also produced on the surface of a probe.

Cavitation—production of gas bubbles at high negative pressure.

Other mechanic effects—radiation power causing streaming in fluids and tension on the contact point of the tissue.

9.1 Thermal effects

When ultrasound beam is transmitted into the tissue, friction power in the tissue makes the ultrasound-induced molecules move, and some energy is absorbed and transformed into heat. Production or loss of heat depends on factors which modify heat production and diffusion. Increased *heat production* is influenced by pressure amplitude of ultrasound, acoustic impedance of tissue, and absorption coefficient of a medium. Diffusion and loss of heat are determined by local tissue perfusion and conduction.

Thermal effect is influenced also by *thermal toleration*. The human body deals with changes of temperature in various physiological processes. To some extent, the body can tolerate them without any further damage. Transformation of absorbed ultrasound into heat depends on the absorption coefficient of the tissue. The highest degree of transformation is typical for the tissues with high absorption coefficient (mainly the bones). On the contrary, the lowest degree of energy transformation takes place in the tissues with low coefficient (e.g., amniotic fluid).

Previous observations have shown that oscillation intensity of 100 mW/cm^2 with frequency of 1 MHz during longitudinal exposure may be the threshold intensity for biological effect of ultrasound. The surface layers are heated in high frequencies, while the deep layers are heated in low frequencies. *Focusation* is considered the most significant factor determining the thermal effects in various oscillation intensities. Focusation controls width of the beam by increase of lateral distribution. As a result, heat production of a medium decreases, and heat distribution becomes more efficient. Finally, it is manifested by decrease of thermal effect [245].

Any adverse effects of the ultrasound have not been described in clinical practice yet. However, this fact cannot be neglected, especially because of increased interest in continual longitudinal monitoring by the transcranial Doppler sonography as well as the more frequent use of color duplex devices in prenatal screening [246].

9.2 Cavitation

The bubbles in body fluids are produced and moved by the ultrasound. There are two types of cavitation: long-term (stable, inert) and temporary (noninert).

Stable cavitation is of great potential to damage the tissue. Bubble are compressing and enlarging continuously. Their size remains the same when shifts of compressions and enlargement are regular. The inert bubble absorbs part of oscillation energy, which will be transformed into heat or circular oscillation. It enables flow of fluids around the bubble, which is followed by pressure effect. Pressure effect may manifest by fragmentation of the cell membranes and biomacromolecules.

Temporary cavitation occurs in bubble oscillation, when the effect of expansion is greater than compression. This increases size of a bubble. Exceeding critical size leads to sudden collapse and occurrence of critical pressure, the so-called shock waves. Intensive increase of pressure and temperature during collapse of bubbles may result from various biological effects such as lysis of the cells, production of free oxygen radicals, and vaporization. Production of free radicals may lead to cell damage. Furthermore, the mutagenous effect is also possible to happen [247]. The Bioeffect Committee of the American Institute of Ultrasound in Medicine [246] states that temporary cavitation may occur in the soft tissues when there are extremely short pulses with power of 3300 W/cm^2. However, it is not reached in the common ultrasound diagnostic process. In recent years, requirements on sonography devices have been increasing as well as power output of the device. Therefore, this effect needs to be taken into consideration in the future.

Results of some studies on animals claim that ultrasound-induced cavitation causes hemorrhage in the lungs and the intestines. These effects have been found in the tissues which were in contact with gas [248–252]. The use of a contrast substance leads to production of microbubbles which provides gas cores for onset of cavitation. This means that the contrast substance decreases the threshold for onset of cavitation.

9.3 Other mechanic effects

The course of ultrasound oscillation causes low-frequency radiation in the tissue. *Radiation* produces pressure in the direction of a bundle of rays from the probe. It should not be confused with oscillation pressure of the ultrasound as such. Pressure and pressure gradient, which are produced in a bundle of rays, are very low, even at higher intensities of a diagnostic range of ultrasound oscillations [253]. The effect of radiation manifests when liquids are present. Oscillation, which may manifest with liquid flow, is produced. The velocity of liquid flow is low, and usually it does not cause any harm.

10. Doppler sonography

In 1842, Austrian physicist *Johann Christian Doppler* (*1803–1853*) in his work called *Über das farbige Licht der Doppelsterne und einiger andere Gestirne des Himmels* described the principle that says that frequency of oscillation changes if the source moves against the observer (**Figure 30**). Doppler's discovery of change of oscillation from a movable source was far ahead of his time. It was applied in practice for the first time in the 1920s. According to the frequency moves recorded in spectral lines of radiation, which come from distant galaxies, for the first time, the astronomers could claim that the universe is enlarging. This discovery, made by Edwin P. Hubble in 1929, has changed significantly the approach of a modern astronomy to nature of the universe [41].

Doppler's effect enabled construction of navigation systems and radars during World War II.

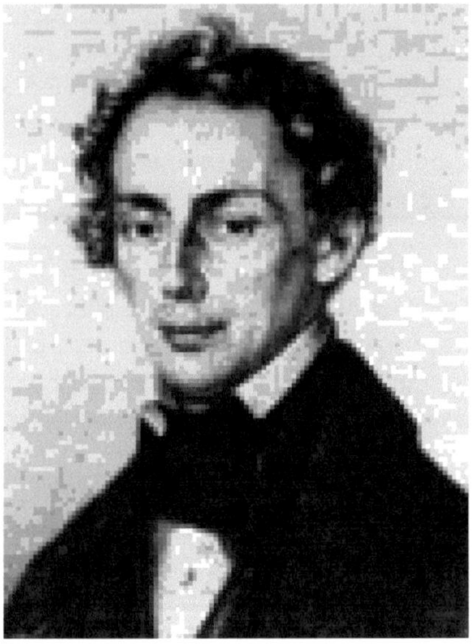

Figure 30.
Johann Christian Doppler (1803–1853). Source: [254].

In medicine, Doppler ultrasonography has been applied just a few decades ago. It was used later than the ultrasound monitoring devices, which were more difficult to construct. In the 1970s, the use of duplex technique has enabled imaging blood flow in the vessel which could be seen in the tomographic B-image. This improved the use of Doppler sonography. Later, modernization of the ultrasound devices has allowed the use of color Doppler imaging in clinical practice. The imaging method based on the Doppler effect is accurate, noninvasive, and accessible. The Doppler effect is a basic principle of the ultrasound diagnostic procedure. It measures velocity of moving particles in vivo. Evaluation of selected hemodynamic parameters of blood flow in vessels is the most common use of Doppler ultrasound. When Doppler sonography is used, the morphologic information gained by traditional ultrasound imaging is enriched with important information, which is functional in its nature [41].

10.1 The role of Doppler principle in ultrasonography

The Doppler effect occurs when the ultrasound frequency changes due to ultrasound oscillation, which is reflected from a moving obstacle (e.g., blood elements in vessels) (**Figure 31**).

When ultrasound oscillation is reflected from moving blood elements in the vessel, the frequency will change in relation to the angle of beam reflection and velocity and direction of blood flow. According to the direction of the blood element movement, whether it goes toward or away from the source of ultrasound oscillation (a probe), the frequency range can be described as positive or negative (**Figure 32**).

The difference between frequency of transmitted and absorbed oscillation is called the frequency Doppler shift (ΔF). It is defined by the following formula:

$$\Delta F = 2.v.\mathrm{Fe}.\cos\ \alpha/C \tag{1}$$

where ΔF is the frequency Doppler shift, v is the velocity of erythrocytes flow, Fe is the emission frequency wave, α is the angle between the ultrasound beam and the vector of erythrocyte flow, and C is the velocity of ultrasound in tissue

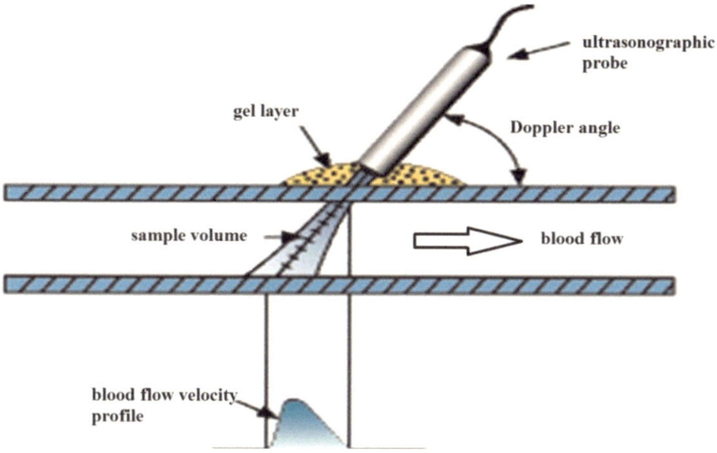

Figure 31.
The Doppler principle.

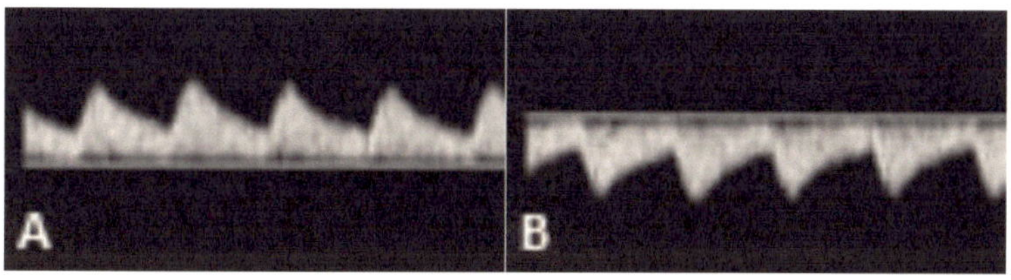

Figure 32.
The Doppler curve of blood flow in the vessel. (A) Blood flow in direction toward the probe, (B) blood flow in direction from the probe.

(it is relatively constant in most tissues of the human body; therefore, the value ΔF is not significantly influenced).

In practice, frequency of ultrasound and velocity of ultrasound wave in tissue is constant. If a constant angle between ultrasound beam and vessel is maintained, velocity of blood flow in the vessel is a determining factor of Doppler frequency shift. The angle of the ultrasound beam and long axis of the vessel is known as *the angle of insonation*. If the angle of insonation is 0°, then frequency shift equals the velocity of blood flow (cos 0° = 1). On the contrary, if the angle of insonation is 90°, then there is no frequency shift. The relation between measured and real velocity of particles can be expressed as $v\ measured = v\ real \times cos\ \alpha$[3]. In theory, the angle of insonation should be as small as possible, but in practice, the beam smaller than 30° is being used. Cos 30° = 0.87 means that measured velocity is 13% smaller than the real velocity.

Two basic types of Doppler record can be distinguished:

- *The spectral record* describes dependence of velocity of blood flow on time and enables determination of flow parameters in the vessel.

- *The color Doppler record* enables to determine direction of blood flow in the vessel and rough range of velocity of blood flow in the vessel.

In the spectral Doppler record, the positive Doppler frequency shifts (flow toward a probe) are drawn above the zero line by red, while the negative frequency shifts (from a probe) are drawn below it by blue (**Figure 32**).

The following *basic Doppler systems* are applied in diagnostic sonography:

- The systems of continuous emission
- The pulsatility systems
- The colorful system of Doppler tomography
- The procedure of color imaging of Doppler power

10.2 The Doppler systems with continuous wave (CW)

The Doppler systems with continuous wave represent the simplest form of Doppler devices. The probes use two piezoelectric elements. One probe transmits ultrasound waves, and the other absorbs reflections of waves continuously. The biggest disadvantage of the system is a lack of axial differentiation. It means that venous structures, which are located in various depths along the axis of the Doppler bundle, are insonated simultaneously and altogether influence the results in the Doppler record. Therefore, it is not possible to determine which part of the total spectrum represents the particular vessel [41].

10.3 The pulsatility Doppler systems (the pulsed waves, PW)

The pulsatility Doppler systems use one piezoelectric element, which transmits and absorbs ultrasound waves alternatively. The probe functions in the alternating regime, which means that after transmitting a short ultrasound impulse, the probe absorbs delayed reflections created in moving blood elements in the vessel.

In the PW method, setting the location and size of sampling volume allows to direct an ultrasound beam to the vessel. The selected size of sampling volume should correspond with the width of transparency in the vessel. If the volume in the middle of the vessel is too low, then the lower frequencies occurring near the vascular wall, where the erythrocytes move slowly, will not be recorded. Therefore, the values of velocity will be significantly increased. On the other hand, when the sampling volume is oversized, measurement takes place in the vessel and its surrounding, the average values will be lower, and high artifact disturbance (noise) will be present [11].

Transmission frequency of oscillation series is called *the pulse repetition frequency* (PRF). The PRF must be at least two times greater than the frequency of detected Doppler shift (the Nyquist's limit) (PRF = 2fdmax). The depth of ultrasound intersection into the tissue decreases due to increasing emission frequency, and thus the PRF has to be the lower, the greater distance between the vessel and the probe is. The PRF values, which are determined by the required depth of intersection, delimit the highest velocity (the Doppler shift), which can be measured [11].

If low PRF is chosen for measuring the velocities, the disturbance artifact, so-called aliasing, occurs. It is manifested by Doppler frequencies lower than ½ PRF in the negative spectrum of values [41] (**Figure 33**).

This phenomenon is responsible for misinformation on frequency shift and causes lower or reverse frequency shift. It is manifested by the signal cutoff and its occurrence on the opposite side of the scale. Therefore, high pulse repetition frequency is necessary for detection of fast moving blood elements caused by high Doppler shift. On the contrary, high frequency controls maximum depth at which the signal can be accepted. It has to be noted that the Doppler shift depends

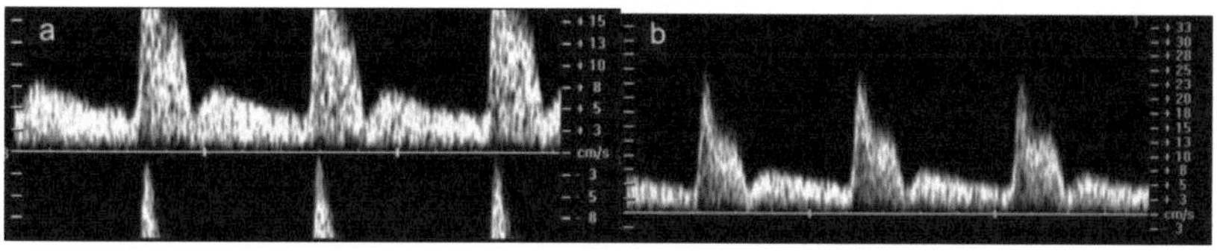

Figure 33.
Aliasing (a) and correction of aliasing (b).

on the transmitter frequency. The relationship between these quantities is as follows [255]:

$$V_{\max} = c^2/8.\text{Fo}.D \tag{2}$$

where V_{max} is the maximum velocity of the moving object (blood elements), c is velocity of ultrasound transmission in the tissue, D is depth at which it is measured, and Fo is frequency of the transmitted signal from the probe.

This relationship shows that the greater the depth for measuring velocity of moving blood cells is, the lower is the maximum detected velocity. That is why blood flow of higher velocity is measured by the low-frequency probes [58, 256].

10.4 The color flow Doppler tomography (CFD, real-time two-dimensional Doppler)

The system of the color Doppler sonography can analyze all Doppler shifts in the selected area. After assessment of the amplitude, frequency, and properties, the CFD transmits echo into the black and color spectra. The B-image is created from the indifferent, nonmoving points. The moving structures, which make the Doppler shift, are drawn by colors. Red color represents the flow toward the probe, blue stands for the flow from the probe, and green is assigned to the turbulent blood flow. The light shades represent fast flow, while the darker ones show slow flow [11, 257].

In neurosonology, the color Doppler sonography is mainly used for accurate detection of strains in the vessel, assessment of blood flow in the sections of vessel, making diagnosis of vascular malformations, and differentiation of the avascular lesions from the vascularized lesions [258–260]. Despite the disadvantages, the color Doppler sonography can in some cases substitute angiography and provides accurate information about vascular structures in the CNS in neonates and infants [261].

10.5 The technique of the color Doppler power mapping (color Doppler energy, CDE; color power angio, CPA; Doppler power mode; power mapping)

The principle of Doppler power mapping is based on determination of the amplitude of Doppler signals created in the moving structures. The color Doppler energy enables better imaging of the tiny vessels with slow blood flow. However, information about the direction and velocity of blood flow is missing here [41]. The advantages of the CDE method are the sensitivity to slow blood flow and independence on the angle of insonation (except of 90°). The three-dimensional reconstructions of anatomy of the blood vessels are more visible in the unified color mapping than in traditional color imagining.

11. The transcranial color-coded Doppler ultrasonography

Transcranial color-coded Doppler ultrasonography (TCCD) enables insonation of the cerebral arteries through the standard acoustic windows. In 1967, Fox was the first to perform the Doppler recording of cerebral arteries [262, 263]. The publication by H. Bada from Springfield, Illinois [264], has been of a great importance for further development. The transcranial Doppler ultrasonography was introduced to clinical medicine by Aaslid [265].

Thanks to the pulse mode, the spectral image is obtained from accurately set distances and simultaneously by color coding from precisely defined segments of the cerebral vessels in two-dimensional imaging and color imaging.

11.1 The transcranial color-coded Doppler ultrasonographic examination

In order to avoid waking or upsetting the child, the examination has to be performed as carefully as possible. The patient should be calm. The lumen of cerebral vessels should be stable, and the position of sample volume in the vessel should be constant. The venous outflow might be decreased, and the real values of the Doppler curve might be changed if the baby's head is rotated inappropriately.

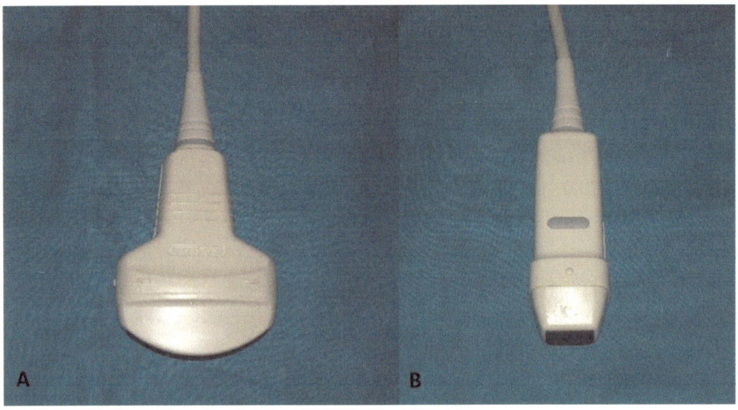

Figure 34.
Sonographic probes. (A) Convex, (B) linear.

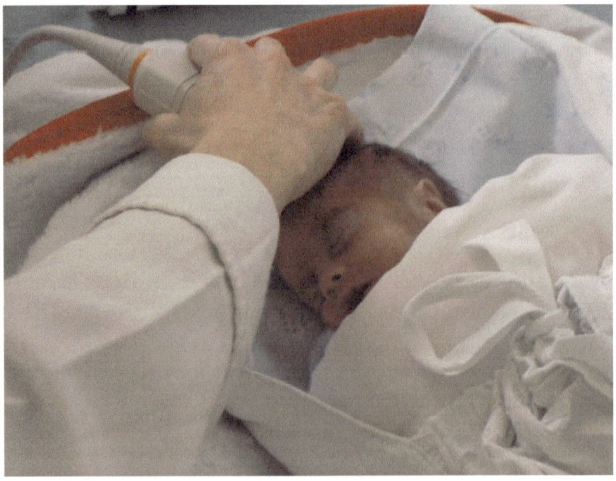

Figure 35.
Examination of a neonate by the transcranial Doppler ultrasonography through the anterior fontanelle.

During examination, it is important to perform the selected method precisely. The double screen for the B real-time image with color-coded flow and the PW image is used. Color coding is used to localize a particular segment of the cerebral vessel and detect direction of blood flow. Appropriate correction of the angle of insonation is of a great importance. The best Doppler signal image containing at least three up to seven cardiac cycles is used for assessment. The measurements are performed by the software equipment. The linear and convex sonographic probes are applied during examination (**Figure 34**) [58, 266].

The following ultrasound approaches can be applied:

- *The approach through the anterior fontanelle* is applied in neonates and infants with the unclosed fontanelle. The probe is placed on the anterior fontanelle in the midline area (**Figure 35**). This approach is mainly used for blood flow imaging in the ACA, ICA, and BA.

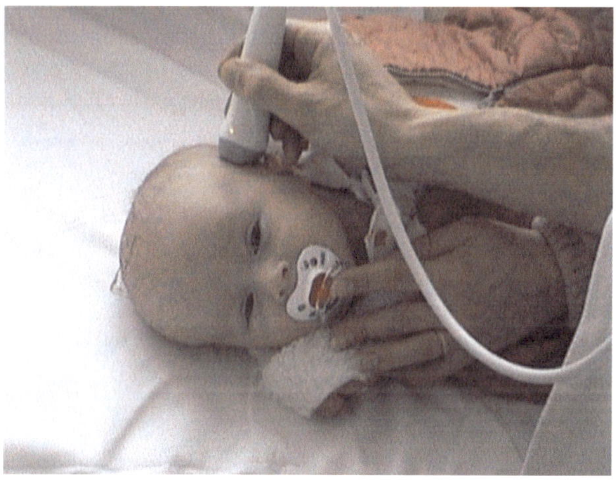

Figure 36.
Examination of the infant by the transcranial Doppler ultrasonography applying the transtemporal approach.

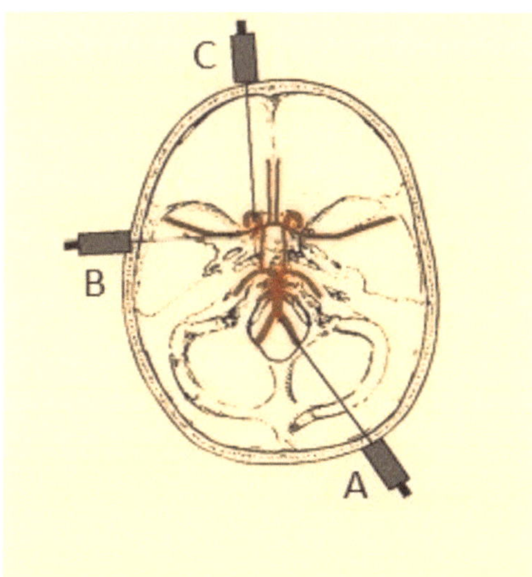

Figure 37.
The transcranial sonographic examinations. (A) The suboccipital approach, (B) the transtemporal approach, (C) the transorbital approach. Adapted from [267].

- *The transtemporal approach* is used to assess blood flow in the MCA and PCA. The probe is introduced into the darkest place on the temporal bone above the zygomatic arch, 1–2 cm from the external auditory canal (**Figures 36** and **37**) [58].
- *The suboccipital approach*—the distal segments of vertebral arteries and basilar artery can be easily visualized through the foramen occipitale magnum (**Figure 37**).
- *The transorbital and submandibular approach* are used occasionally (**Figure 37**).
- *The approach through the defects of calva* (posttraumatic, postsurgical).

During examination, firstly, *the basal Doppler parameters* are assessed by a sonographic probe, which touches the skin gently through the layer of a gel. Then *the compressive test on the anterior fontanelle* is carried out. The Doppler parameters are assessed, while the anterior fontanelle is compressed by the sonographic probe or ophthalmodynamometer. The pressure is stated in g/cm^2 (**Figure 38**). Measurement is performed through the anterior fontanelle or the temporal acoustic window [269–271]. The compressive test on the anterior fontanelle is considered positive if the basal RI value of cerebral vessels increases more than 25% or the value of compressive RI is higher than 0.90 [271].

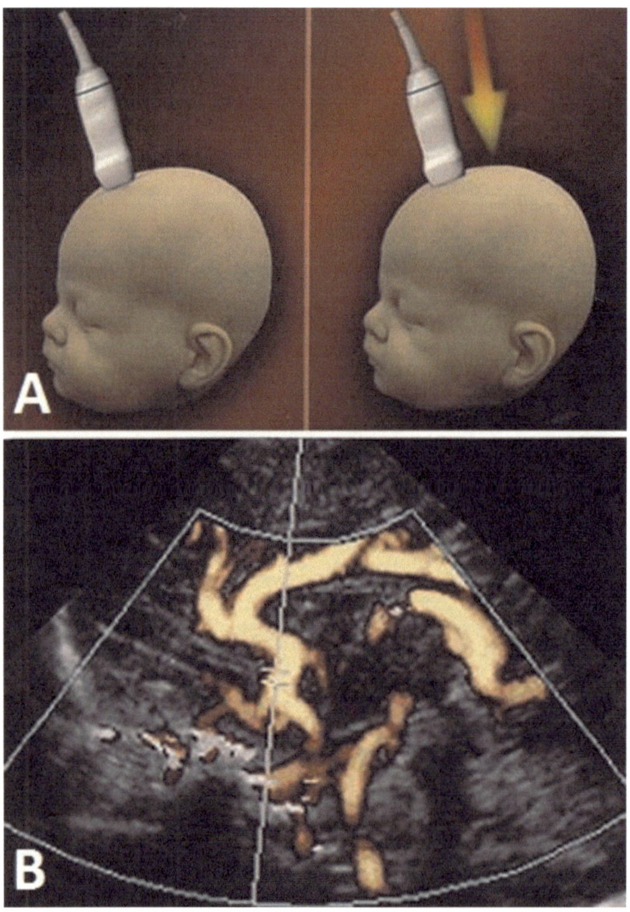

Figure 38.
The compression test on the anterior fontanelle. (A) Compression by the sonographic probe, (B) the Doppler curve of the anterior cerebral artery [268].

DOI: http://dx.doi.org/10.5772/intechopen.89067

12. The Doppler curve, measured and calculated parameters

12.1 The Doppler curve

The cerebral circulation is a low-resistance vascular system, which is typical for organs requiring constant high minute blood flow. The Doppler curve of low-resistance vascular circulation is characterized by positive blood flow during systole but also during diastole (**Figures 39** and **40**). In contrast, the physiological process of a high-resistance vascular system Doppler curve, for example, in the extremities,

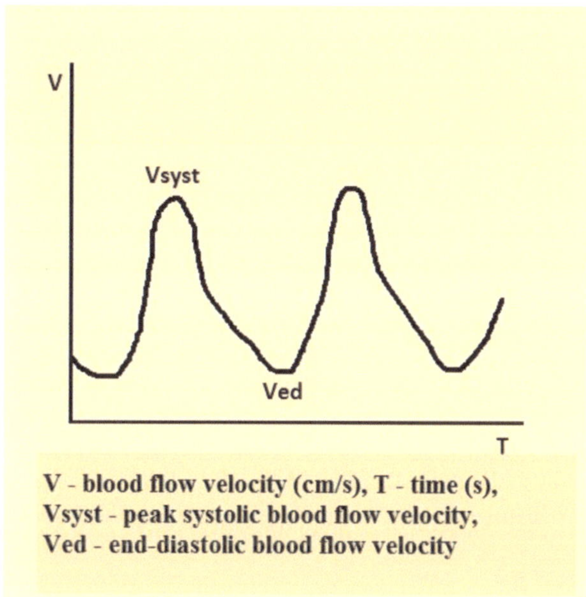

Figure 39.
The schematic diagram of the Doppler curve blood flow in the cerebral artery.

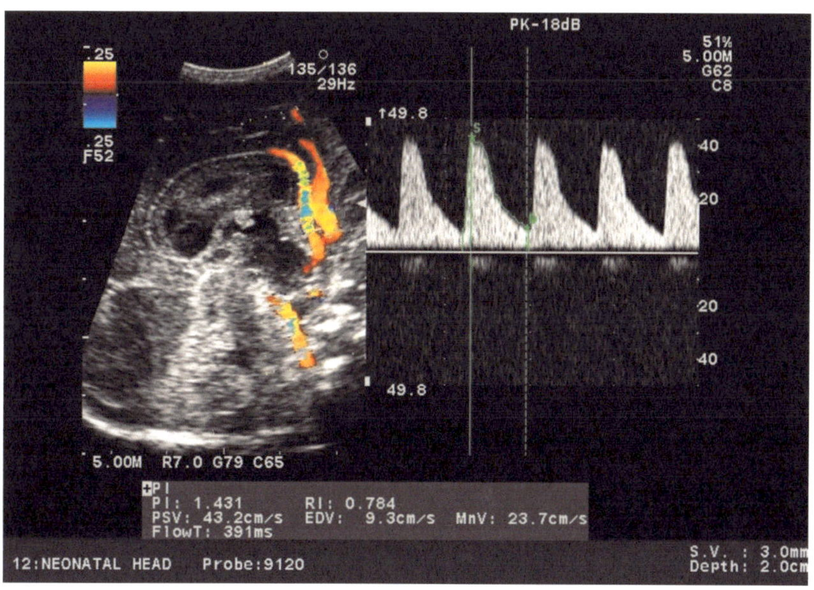

Figure 40.
The Doppler curve of blood flow in the anterior cerebral artery (the low-resistive vascular network).

has three phases and is characterized by short-term reverse flow during early diastole and short positive flow during end-diastole (**Figure 41**) [242].

In physiologic conditions, blood flow is laminar in its nature. The highest velocity is in the middle, while the lowest is near the vascular wall. When pressure gradient rapidly increases during systole, blood flow in the arterial network increases, too. Therefore, systolic segment of the Doppler curve is characterized by rapid increase. During diastole, blood flow decreases, and thus erythrocytes near the vascular wall move slower than erythrocytes which are in the middle of the vessel. Therefore, the diastolic phase of the spectrum is lower; its profile is nonhomogeneous and rich in various frequency shifts.

The shape of the arterial Doppler curve is influenced by various factors. Myocardial contraction creates pressure gradient in the arterial network. Rapid increase of systolic segment of the curve depends on a range of pressure gradients, vascular wall elasticities, and blood viscosities. The pressure wave diminishes in distal direction, and thus velocity of blood flow decreases. Myocardial contraction transfers energy into the elastic vascular wall of the great arteries. Their gradual compression during diastolic phase of the pulse wave ensures continuous prograde blood flow. Blood flow decreases during diastole. The shape and properties of diastolic phase of the Doppler curve are characterized primarily by resistance of the distal vascular network and secondarily by systemic, venous, and intrathoracic pressure. When peripheral vascular resistance is high, velocity of diastolic blood flow decreases. Sometimes it can even drop down to negative values. In physiological conditions, diastolic blood flow in cerebral arteries has always the same direction as the systolic [11].

12.2 Measured and assessed parameters of the Doppler curve

The following parameters can be assessed by the Doppler curve of blood flow in cerebral arteries:

Peak systolic blood flow velocity (*Vsyst*)—the maximal velocity pulse wave. The value is expressed by maximal height of the curve during systole.

End-diastolic blood flow velocity (Ved)—the value of end-diastole is assessed instead of the minimal blood flow velocity during diastole.

Mean blood flow velocity (Vmean)—it expresses the value of mean blood flow velocity between the beginning of systole and end of diastole during one cardiac cycle. Blood flow velocity is stated in cm/s or m/s.

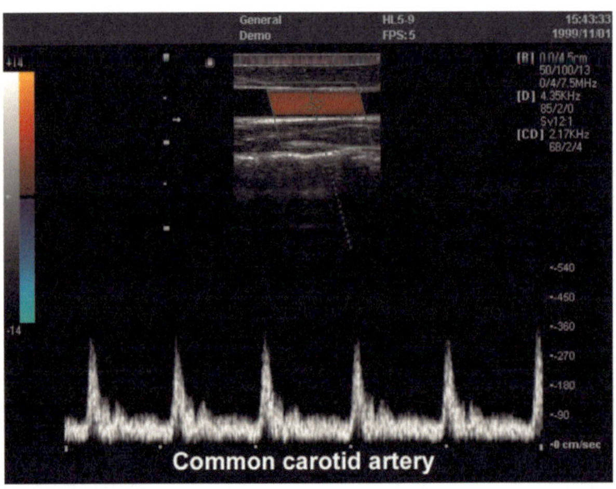

Figure 41.
The Doppler curve of blood flow in common carotid artery (the high-resistance vascular network).

From the aspect of cerebral perfusion assessment, the assessment of systolic and diastolic velocities from blood flow is not sufficient, because the values are very variable. Concerning change in vessel caliber, the change in blood flow velocity does not have to correspond with the change in degree of perfusion [272]. This deficit can be substituted by qualitative analysis of the Doppler curve, which compares systolic and diastolic blood flow velocities in the vessel [273].

The advantage of qualitative analysis of the Doppler curve is the fact that the results are less influenced by the nonstandard angle α and local turbulences in the arterial lumen. The angle of insonation has impact on systolic and diastolic velocities, but the ratio of velocities remains stable.

The most common indices of the Doppler curve are as follows:

The resistance index (*RI, Pourcelot index*) has been used in 1974. It is a parameter showing resistance of the vascular network. It is defined as:

$$RI = Vsyst\text{–}Ved/Vsyst \tag{3}$$

The pulsatility index (PI, Gösling index) is defined by Gösling in 1969:

$$PI = Vsyst\text{–}Ved/Vmean \tag{4}$$

Regarding the mean blood flow velocity, the PI values in a place of a denominator are higher than the RI values. PI is very important especially in zero or retrograde diastolic blood flow when RI or S/D index cannot be calculated [274].

The *systolic-diastolic ratio (S/D index) is defined as:*

$$S/D = Vsyst/Ved \tag{5}$$

Another parameter of the Doppler curve is the acceleration time (AT), which is measured from the beginning of systole until it reaches the maximal velocity [275]. It is determined by the factors such as myocardial contractibility, cardiac output, arterial blood pressure, and vessel compliance.

12.3 Development of Doppler parameters of cerebral circulation: physiological values

The normal values of blood flow velocity in cerebral vessels, which can be assessed by transcranial Doppler ultrasonography in adults [276–282] and children [37, 278, 283–287], have been published repeatedly.

In order to differentiate of pathological values, knowledge of the physiological range of values is an inevitable background of an examining method. Although the parameters of cerebral circulation examined by Doppler technique have been published repeatedly, there are no unified and generally accepted reference values. The issue of normal values is caused by several reasons:

- Use of various ultrasonographical equipment
- Developmental changes in quality of Doppler equipment
- Unknown technical parameters and methodology
- Nonunified documentation and presentation of results

The reference values published by the authors stated above are not generally applicable. In the Clinic of Neurosurgery at the University Hospital Martin, we use physiological values proposed by Minárik [58] with precisely defined methodology and examination technique. The values of selected parameters of the Doppler curve of cerebral arteries are shown in **Tables 6–8**. The critical RI values are those which are increased at a maximum of about 0.05 in comparison with the utmost value of a normal range.

12.3.1 Neonates

During the first three weeks of life, the linear correlation between age and blood flow velocity in cerebral arteries is being observed. As they are getting older, the blood flow velocity increases in all cerebral arteries. The degree of blood flow increase throughout cerebral arteries does not depend on weight and gaining weight. The most significant changes occur in the first hours and days after birth because increase of blood flow velocity in cerebral arteries and decrease of

	1st month	1st month	3rd month	3rd month	6th month	6th month	12th month	12th month
	A1	A3	A1	A3	A1	A3	A1	A3
Vsyst	67–82	56–69	74–87	64–77	81–90	68–85	95–104	87–96
Ved	19–28	18–27	21–34	20–31	26–34	25–33	25–44	33–40
Vmean	36–46	29–42	36–54	30–50	46–58	38–54	57–67	51–63
RI	0.65–0.73	0.60–0.69	0.59–0.71	0.59–0.69	0.62–0.68	0.58–0.65	0.57–0.63	0.58–0.62

Table 6.
Reference values of parameters of the Doppler curve of the anterior cerebral artery (arterial segments A1 and A3) in months [58].

	1st month	1st month	3rd month	3rd month	6th month	6th month	12th month	12th month
	M1	M3	M1	M3	M1	M3	M1	M3
Vsyst	75–86	65–80	80–90	70–79	91–100	83–92	104–115	95–106
Ved	20–30	19–28	24–35	22–32	32–40	28–36	41–49	36–45
Vmean	39–51	35–49	46–60	41–55	56–68	51–65	64–80	61–74
RI	0.65–0.74	0.63–0.73	0.61–0.70	0.60–0.70	0.60–0.65	0.59–0.66	0.55–0.61	0.56–0.62

Table 7.
Reference values of parameters of the Doppler curve of the right middle cerebral artery (arterial segments M1 and M3) in months [58].

	1st month	1st month	3rd month	3rd month	6th month	6th month	12th month	12th month
	M1	M3	M1	M3	M1	M3	M1	M3
Vsyst	75–85	64–79	80–90	70–82	91–99	81–90	103–112	96–106
Ved	20–29	19–28	23–34	22–30	32–40	29–37	41–48	38–45
Vmean	39–51	35–49	48–62	40–56	57–68	50–66	64–80	57–72
RI	0.65–0.73	0.62–0.71	0,63–0.68	0.60–0.68	0.59–0.65	0.56–0.68	0.56–0.61	0.57–0.64

Table 8.
Reference values of parameters of the Doppler curve of left middle cerebral artery (arterial segments M1 and M3) in months [58].

The standard values of the basal RI-ACA in the segment before genu corporis callosi in preterm neonates	
<33rd gestation week	0.77 ± 0.09
>34th gestation week	0.70 ± 0.07

Table 9.
The standard values of the Doppler curve resistance index of ACA in the segment before genu corporis callosi in preterm neonates [271, 284].

resistance index are very rapid. Generally, preterm neonates have lower blood flow velocity reflected in higher value of resistance index (**Table 9**). Higher degree of immaturity and lower weight at birth are linked with higher percentage of changes in Ved. In hypotrophic neonates, decreased Vsyst and Vmean were observed in the anterior cerebral artery, but blood flow velocity in the middle cerebral artery did not change. The Doppler parameters of cerebral arteries in hypotrophic neonates are influenced by weight at birth, gestational age, and mother's smoking during pregnancy due to intrauterine growth retardation [288].

12.3.2 Infancy

After the third week of age, increase of blood flow velocity in cerebral arteries slows down. The maximal values are reached before the age of 9 years. Since then blood flow velocity gradually decreases in an average of about 1–1.5 cm/s/year. The values for adults are reached in the age of 18 years. The resistance index gradually decreases during 12 months of age from the value of 0.70 to the value of 0.55 and then remains the same. In physiological conditions, blood flow velocity measured in the right and left parts of the brain does not change significantly [58].

12.4 The factors influencing the value of qualitative indices of the Doppler curve

The values of qualitative indices of the Doppler curve of blood flow are influenced mainly by the factors which change the diastolic segment of the curve. An overview of extra- and intracranial factors, which have impact on the Doppler parameters of the cerebral arteries, is shown in **Table 10**. During examination, the factors described below need to be taken into consideration as well:

- *Interindividual norms*. Methodology applied in measurement and technical parameters of ultrasound equipment have to be taken in account. When the results are ambiguous, it is recommended to observe dynamic intraindividual trends instead of comparing measured values with the norm [11, 58].

- *Physical and mental activity* can also influence cerebral perfusion. During increased mental and physical activity of infants and older children, systolic, diastolic, and mean blood flow velocities in the proximal and distal segments of arteries have been significantly increased in the observed cerebral arteries. However, the resistance index did not change significantly if activity was changed [58].

- *Manipulation with the neonate, moving him from the incubator to a bed, and endotracheal suction from cannula* may increase blood flow velocity in cerebral arteries as well.

- Taking higher amount of blood sample, bradycardia, and apneic pauses may lead to decreased cerebral blood circulation, too.

12.4.1 The factors increasing the resistance index of cerebral arteries

- *Acute intracranial hypertension* accompanies brain injuries, brain edema, and active hydrocephalus. It is manifested by increased RI and decreased, zero, or even reverse blood flow during diastole. The Vsyst values do not change significantly.

- *Hypocapnia*—decrease of p_aCO_2 causes vasoconstriction of cerebral arteries, and thus cerebral blood flow decreases. Decrease of p_aCO_2 results in decrease of Ved and increase of RI. Rapid decrease of p_aCO_2 leads to decrease of Vsyst [290]. Loss of vascular reactivity to change of p_aCO_2 is in relatively good correlation with severity and prognosis of child's clinical condition [291].

Hyperoxia—increased p_aO_2 causes mild vasoconstriction of cerebral arteries and is linked to decreased cerebral blood flow. The cerebrovascular response to change of p_aO_2 is more uniform than the response to p_aCO_2.

Congenital heart disease with left-to-right short circuit, for example, ductus arteriosus Botalli persistens truncus arteriosus, can have negative impact on cerebral perfusion. The range of changes in cerebral circulation depends on hemodynamic severity of left-to-right short circuit. No changes in the Doppler curve can be observed in small-signal short circuit [292, 293].

Indomethacin induces vasoconstrictions of cerebral arteries. The use of indomethacin increases resistance index of cerebral arteries. Inadequately high doses of indomethacin may cause ischemic damage of cerebral tissue.

Blood hyperviscosity—in polyglobulia, it is accompanied by decrease of absolute values of blood flow velocity in cerebral arteries and just mild increase of resistance index. Changes can occur in proximal and distal segments of cerebral arteries. Changes of the Doppler curve parameters during change of hematocrit are influenced by changes of viscosity and rheological properties of blood.

In *intraventricular hemorrhage* in neonates, increase of RI and decrease of Ved occur in cerebral arteries on the site of hemorrhage. But change is mild or none in arteries, in which branches do not protrude into the site of hemorrhage or do so only partially. The range of changes of parameters of the Doppler blood flow curve

	Extracranial factors	**Intracranial factors**
Increased resistance index	Hypocapnia, hyperoxia, congenital heart disease with left-to-right short circuit (ductus arteriosus Botalli persistens, truncus arteriosus), polyglobulia, blood hyperviscosity, increased hematocrit, indomethacin, severe arterial hypotension, decreased cardiac output, neuronal death	Acute intracranial hypertension (brain injury, cerebral edema, active hydrocephalus), brain infarction, intracerebral and intraventricular hemorrhage
Decreased resistance index	Hypercapnia, hypoxemia, hypoxia, seizures, asphyxia, hyaline membrane disease, increased cardiac output, hypervolemia, increased central venous pressure (right-sided heart failure, pneumothorax)	Inflammatory congestion, arteriovenous malformations of the brain, seizures

Table 10.
Extracranial and intracranial factors influencing the Doppler parameters of cerebral arteries [289].

depends on severity of IVH and accompanying factors. In IVH of grades 3 and 4, changes can be detected in all main cerebral vessels [58, 264].

In *severe systemic arterial hypotension*, resistance index of cerebral arteries increases due to significant decrease of blood flow velocity during diastole in low cardiac output.

In determination of *neuronal death*, prograde diastolic blood flow in cerebral arteries cannot be seen.

Brain infarction—usually after acute brain infarction, blood flow is not initially detectable in a particular segment, and decreased Ved with increased RI is detected in proximal segment of the vessel. Arterial recanalization can be detected by gradual return of the Doppler signal to the standard curve followed by temporary increase of velocity, probably a sign of hyperemia [58, 278].

12.4.2 Factors decreasing the resistance index of cerebral arteries

Hypercapnia causes vasodilatation of cerebral arteries and increases blood flow in the brain. When p_aCO_2 increases, Ved increases but RI decreases. When increase of p_aCO_2 is more rapid, Vsyst increases, too.

Hypoxia—decrease of p_aO_2 has strong vasodilatation effect, which can suppress vasoconstriction effect of hypocapnia in standard conditions [294, 295].

Seizures decrease resistance index of cerebral arteries. Increased metabolic demands of the brain give rise to vasodilatation.

Inflammatory congestion decreases the resistance index. But the index increases during progression of hyperemia and development of intracranial hypertension.

Asphyxia—immediately after asphyxia, the values of resistance index of cerebral arteries can be abnormal, determined by moderate redistribution of blood circulation, cardiac output, and cerebral autoregulation. Afterward, postasphyctic cerebral hyperemia, characterized by the so-called soft flow with high values of blood flow velocity during diastole and low resistance index, occurs [296].

Hyaline membrane disease (*idiopathic respiratory distress syndrome, IRDS*) is a combination of hypoxia, hypercapnia, and systemic arterial hypotension. If autoregulatory mechanisms of cerebral circulation are functional, the resistance index of cerebral arteries can get back to normal by adequate ventilation regime [11, 297].

In *increased cardiac output* or in *hypervolemia*, the resistance index usually decreases.

Conditions with *increased central venous pressure*, for example, pneumothorax, endotracheal suction from cannula, and right-sided heart failure, result in decrease of resistance index of cerebral vessels.

In *venous anomalies of the brain*, bidirectional flows are often present, but also steal phenomenon may occur.

13. Morphology of the cerebral ventricles in pediatric hydrocephalus

For the reason of difficult accessibility, assessment of volume of the cerebral ventricles by computed analysis is not commonly used in children with hydrocephalus in clinical practice. Linear morphometric parameters, which can precisely detect intracranial structures, are preferred instead. Assessment of morphology of CSF pathways by USG, CT, or MRI examination plays a crucial role in assessment of dynamics of pediatric hydrocephalus.

Considering detection of onset of the cerebral ventricle dilatation and further observation of its dynamics in neonates and infants with hydrocephalus (before closure of the anterior fontanelle), *transcranial ultrasonography* plays the most important role [298, 299]. Gyrification of the brain, shift of midline structures, the CSF pathways (the cerebral ventricles and subarachnoid space), and pathological lesions are assessed by ultrasonography. Transcranial ultrasonography enables assessment of dynamics of intracranial bleeding in preterm neonates. In acute hydrocephalus, dilatation and roundness of the occipital and temporal horns of the lateral cerebral ventricles and the trigonum area develop at first. Especially the frontal horns and bodies of the lateral cerebral ventricles are enlarged in ventriculomegaly due to cerebral atrophy [11].

In a child with hydrocephalus, *morphometry of the cerebral ventricles and subarachnoid space* is an important part of the ultrasonographic examination. Accurate size of the CSF pathways enables comparison with standard values as well as observation of intraindividual dynamics. Subjective assessment of the CSF pathways should be done together with size measurement. The most common morphologic parameters of the brain measured in children with hydrocephalus are as follows:

- Wdx.—width of the right lateral cerebral ventricle (usually width of the frontal horn in the coronal plane going through the foramen of Monro)
- Wsin.—width of the left lateral cerebral ventricle
- VIdx.—ventricular index of the right lateral cerebral ventricle (the ventricular index, the greatest distance of the lateral wall of the anterior horn of the lateral cerebral ventricle from midline)
- VIsin—ventricular index of the left lateral cerebral ventricle, size of the third and fourth cerebral ventricles, width of the interhemispheric fissure, and width of the subarachnoid spaces on convexity
- IV—interventricular distance (distance between the lateral corners of the lateral cerebral ventricles)
- TC—transcerebral size (width of both hemispheres)
- Thickness of the cortical mantle (**Figure 42**)

The frontal and temporal horn ratio (the ratio of interventricular distance between the frontal and temporal horns of the lateral cerebral ventricles) is probably the new ultrasonographic index, which can be easily measured on the coronal sonographic section of the brain. The statistical comparison between new frontal and temporal horn ratio and commonly used frontal and occipital horn ratio shows strong linear correlation between both coefficients [300].

Many researchers have dealt with determination of the reference values for assessment of size of the cerebral ventricles in neonates by transcranial ultrasonography. Davies et al. [301] measured the reference values of linear size of the cerebral ventricles in preterm neonates between 23rd and 33rd gestation week (**Table 11**). The size of the frontal horn of the lateral cerebral ventricle corresponded with results of the research by Perry et al. [302]. They determined the value of 3 mm as the upper limit for the 26th–42nd gestational week. The values of thalamo-occipital distance were similar to the fetal values in this gestation age [303]. The position of the head during examination and gender of a child did not have impact on the value

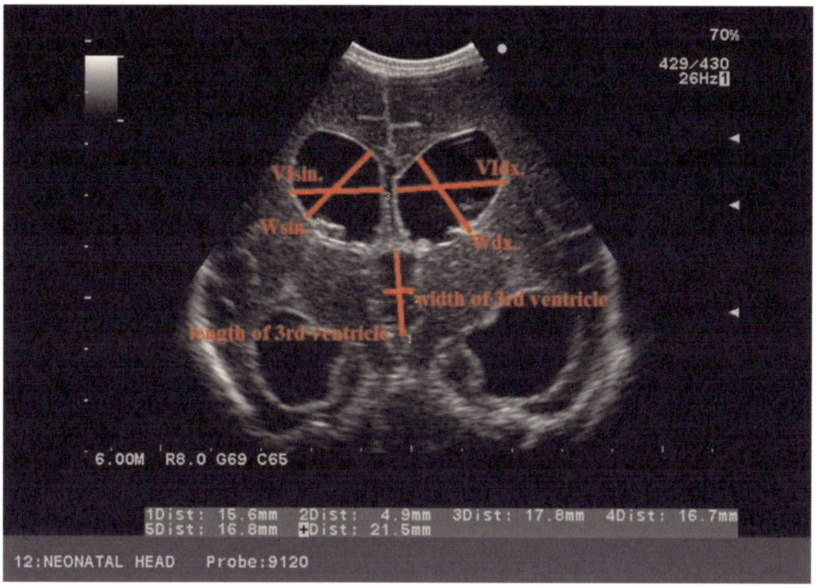

Figure 42.
Examination of the brain of a neonate by transcranial ultrasonography—morphometry of the cerebral ventricles.

The linear parameters of cerebral ventricles	Mean	SD	Referential scale
Width of the frontal horn of the lateral cerebral ventricle	1.27	0.81	0–2.9
Thalamo-occipital distance	16.7	4.0	8.7–24.7
Width of the third cerebral ventricle	1.07	0.74	0–2.6
Width of the fourth cerebral ventricle	5.37	1.03	3.3–7.4
Length of the fourth cerebral ventricle	4.74	1.09	2.6–6.9

Table 11.
The reference values of linear parameters of the cerebral ventricles in preterm neonates between 23rd and 33rd gestation weeks measured by transcranial ultrasonography [301].

of parameters measured. The highest variability, but in acceptable low values, was found in the size of the fourth cerebral ventricle. Perry et al. [302] confirmed that width of the frontal horn of the lateral cerebral ventricle does not change between 26th and 42nd gestation week. Similarly, Sauerbrei et al. [304] found out that ventricular index does not change between 25th and 35th gestation week.

On the other side, results of other research on assessment of size of the cerebral ventricles in a wide range of gestational ages confirmed that ventricular index of the frontal horn of the lateral cerebral ventricle slightly increases regarding gestational age of the infant (**Figures 43** and **44**) [305, 306]. Sondhi et al. [307] also confirmed a slight increase of size of the cerebral ventricles (size of the frontal horn of the lateral cerebral ventricle, thalamo-occipital distance, and width of the third and fourth cerebral ventricle) in relation to gestational age of the infant. But it was proportional to change of the brain tissue.

The *computed tomography* (*CT*) or *nuclear magnetic resonance* (*MRI*) is used for a more precise assessment of the intracranial morphology. Beam radiation, which has a negative effect on a child's organism, is the main disadvantage of CT examination. When these examination techniques are indicated, transport of the child, especially in nonstable preterm neonates, and necessity of sedation have to be taken into consideration. Active hydrocephalus can be detected by the presence of typical

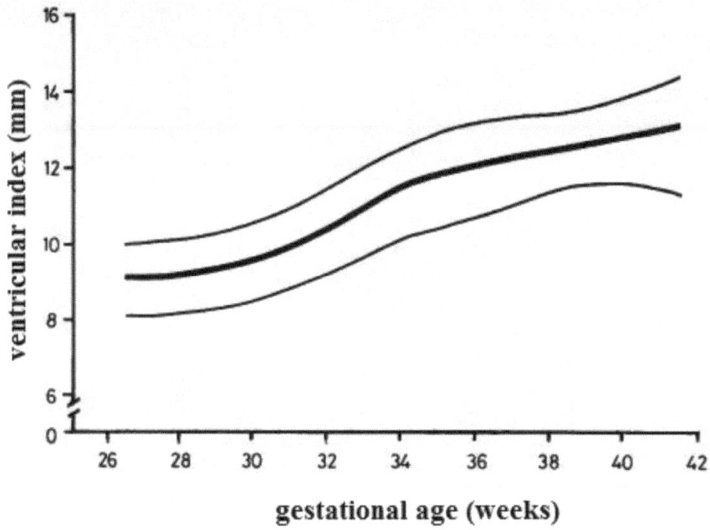

Figure 43.
The values of ventricular index in neonates in relationship to gestational age (adapted from [305]). The upper and lower line shows the 3rd and 97th percentile. Ventricular index, the greatest horizontal distance between the lateral wall of the frontal horn of the lateral cerebral ventricle and midline.

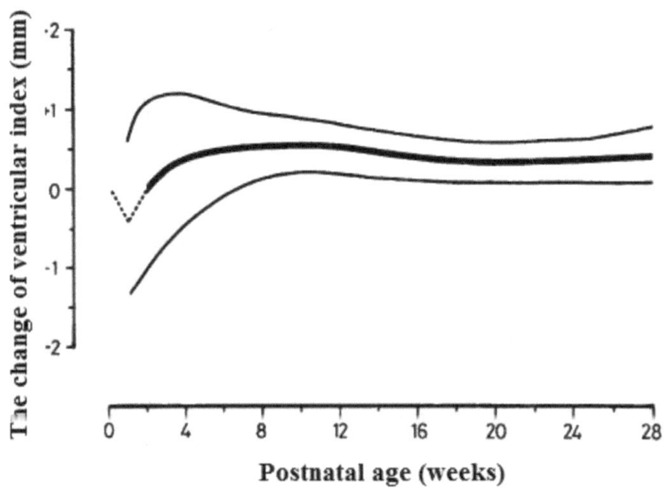

Figure 44.
Change of ventricular index of the cerebral ventricles in neonates and infants in relation to postnatal age (adapted from [305]). The upper and lower line shows the 3rd and 97th percentile. Ventricular index, the greatest horizontal distance between the lateral wall of the frontal horn of the lateral cerebral ventricle and midline.

periventricular hypodensity or increased intensity of the signal in T2-weighted MRI image due to transependymal diffusion of cerebrospinal fluid (**Figure 6**). In pathological lesions, MRI technique enables accurate measurement of degree and relation to the surrounding structures. Degree of hypoxic-ischemic brain damage can be also clearly seen in an MRI image. Flow of cerebrospinal fluid through CSF pathways can be shown by cine-phase MRI sequence. It is also used in postsurgical assessment of the function of endoscopic ventriculostomy of the third cerebral ventricle (**Figure 45**). The combination of CT or MRI examination with neuronavigation enables to plan trajectory and depth of ventricular catheter insertion of drainage systems and precise insertion of neuroendoscope into the cerebral ventricles (**Figure 46**) [189].

Width of the frontal horn of the lateral cerebral ventricle in the coronal plane; sonographic section through the foramen of Monro; thalamo-occipital distance in the parasagittal section, in which whole lateral cerebral ventricle is presented; distance between the thalamus and the most dorsal segment of the occipital horn of the lateral cerebral ventricle; width of the third cerebral ventricle in the axial plane near the foramen of Monro; width and length of the fourth cerebral ventricle between the right and left side of the lateral recess; width and length of the fourth cerebral ventricle in the transverse axis through the posterior aperture, through asterion used as an acoustic window. Width of the fourth cerebral ventricle represents the distance between the base and peak of a triangle. SD, standard deviation.

When morphometry of the CSF pathways is assessed on CT and MRI image, the following linear parameters of the brain are taken into consideration (**Figures 47** and **48**): Evans' index, the ratio between maximum width of the frontal horns of the lateral cerebral ventricles and maximal internal diameter with of the calva [308]; the ratio between the frontal horns of the lateral cerebral ventricles (FHR, frontal horn ratio); the ratio between maximum width of the frontal horns of the lateral cerebral ventricles and maximal internal diameter of the calva at the same level; the bicaudate ratio, the ratio between width of the lateral cerebral ventricles between the caudate nuclei and maximal internal diameter width of the calva at the same level; the ratio between the frontal and occipital horns of the lateral cerebral ventricles (FOR, frontal/occipital horn ratio); and the ratio between sum of maximum width of the frontal and occipital horns of the lateral cerebral ventricles and twice the amount of maximal internal diameter width of the calva [309]. Ventriculomegaly is defined by Evans' index ≥ 0.30. The standard value of FOR equals 0.37, and it is independent on child's age [309].

Interesting results can be found in the research by Eide [310] who assessed the relationship between intracranial pressure and size of the cerebral ventricles in hydrocephalus, craniosynostosis, and dysfunction of drainage systems. To measure

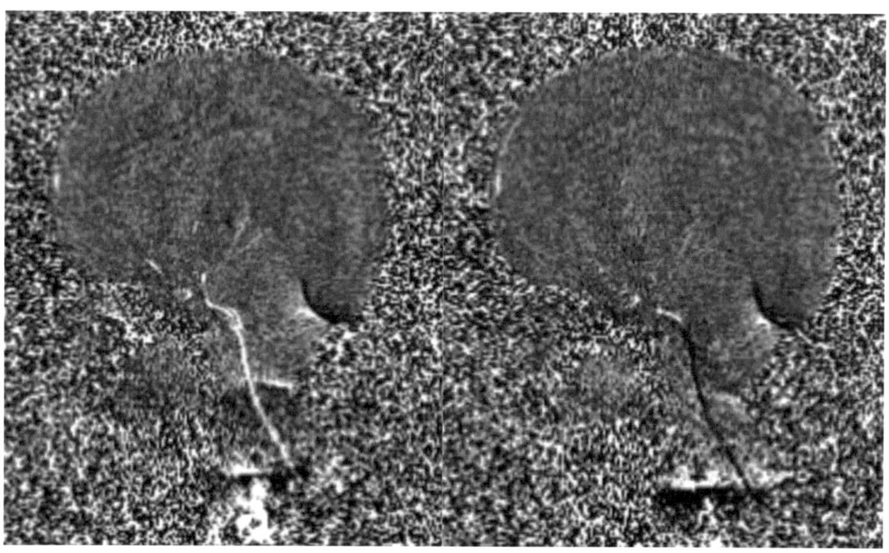

Figure 45.
The cine-phase MRI examination of flow of cerebrospinal fluid through endoscopic third ventriculostomy in the child with hydrocephalus.

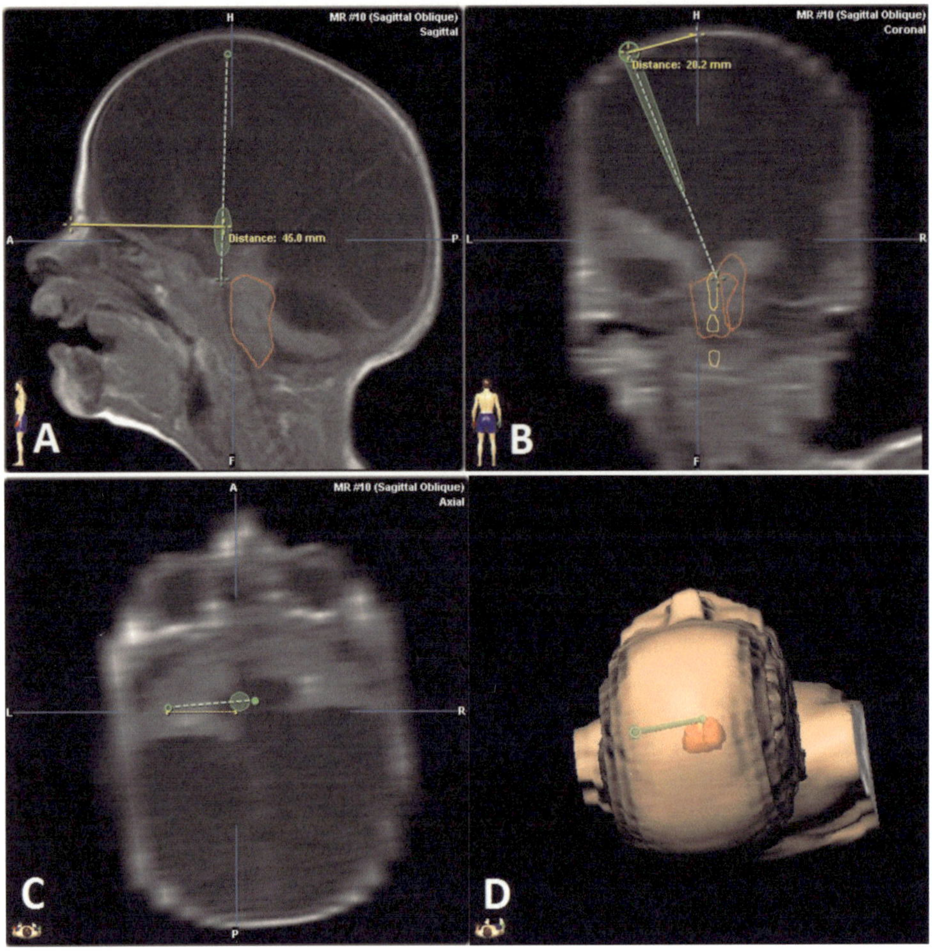

Figure 46.
Planning of trajectory for neuroendoscope before ETV by Brainlab neuronavigation.

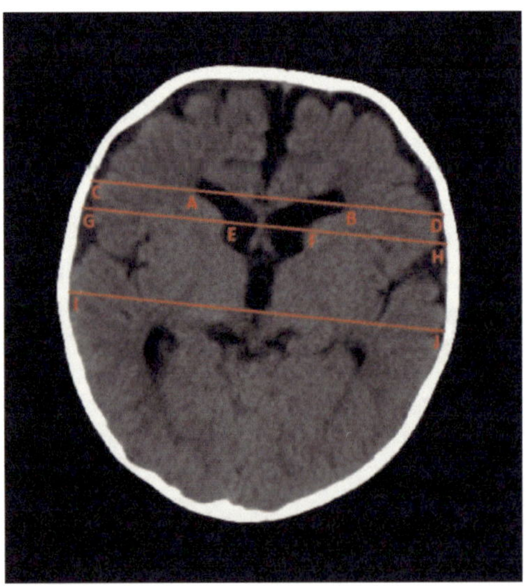

Figure 47.
CT of the brain—the linear morphometric parameters. Evans' index = distance AB/IJ, frontal horn ratio (FHR, ratio between the frontal horns and the lateral cerebral ventricles) = AB/CD, bicaudate ratio = EF/GH.

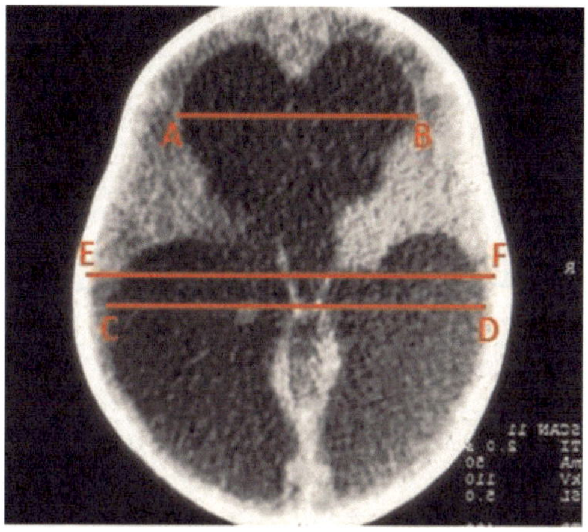

Figure 48.
CT of the brain—FOR measurement (frontal/occipital horn ratio, ratio of the frontal and occipital horns of the lateral cerebral ventricles), FOR = (AB + CD)/2 × EF.

intracranial pressure, he used the continual ICP monitoring with quantitative analysis of the data. The size of the intracranial ventricles was assessed by selected linear morphometric parameters. Significant correlation was not confirmed between current size of the cerebral ventricles and value of intracranial pressure in the sample of 184 patients. The relationship between measured parameters was not influenced by age of patients nor etiology of intracranial hypertension. In addition, statistically significant correlation between long-term change of size of the cerebral ventricles and change of intracranial pressure was not observed either. Statistically significant correlation between change of size of the cerebral ventricles and change of mean of ICP or number of peaks of ICP was not found in 31 cases of simultaneous measurement of ICP and size of the cerebral ventricles. The results show that assessment of current size and long-term change of size of the cerebral ventricles by CT examination, in craniostenosis and dysfunction of the drainage systems, is not a reliable indicator of current value and change of value of intracranial pressure.

Low correlation between size of the cerebral ventricles and pressure of the anterior fontanelle was also confirmed in 19 cases of asymptomatic pediatric hydrocephalus [311]. Statistically significant correlation between size of the cerebral ventricles and change of ICP values was not observed in the sample of 12 cases of asymptomatic intracranial hypertension [312]. Statistically significant correlation between mean of intracranial pressure measured during lumbar puncture and size of the cerebral ventricles measured by CT examination was not found in a bigger sample of 181 children with communicating hydrocephalus [313].

In experimental conditions, a decreased number of structural proteins and enzymes bound to myelin followed by demyelination and axonal loss were measured in the white matter in cases of progressive hydrocephalus [314]. Assessment of changes in the white and gray matter of the brain before and after drainage procedure showed that early drainage of cerebrospinal fluid in progressive pediatric hydrocephalus is the basic requirement for positive neurological outcome of treatment [315].

Volume of the cerebral ventricles in children with hydrocephalus before insertion of drainage system can be up to 14 times the standard value. Gradual decrease of size of the cerebral ventricles can last 6 months *after insertion of the drainage system (shunt)*. Change in amount of volume of the cerebral ventricles can be also influenced by a type of drainage system, especially a valve used. Xenos et al. [316]

confirmed a significant postsurgical decrease of volume of the cerebral ventricles in children with hydrocephalus after insertion of the medium pressure cylindrical valve shunt compared with insertion of the Delta 1.5 valve (Medtronic PS Medical, Goleta, California). However, difference was not confirmed in statistical analysis. Despite that fact, the authors of the study suppose that the medium pressure cylindrical valve shunt can cause hyperdrainage in comparison with the Delta 1.5 valve, especially within first months after operation. Jain et al. [317] confirmed that the first insertion of the medium pressure cylindrical valve shunt decreased size of the cerebral ventricles in comparison to cases with initial insertion of the Delta 1.5 valve. No difference in postsurgical change of size of the cerebral ventricles between these two types of shunts was found when revision of dysfunctional drainage systems had been performed. In children with drainage system, change of size of the cerebral ventricles can change intracranial dynamics, viscoelastic properties, compliance of the brain tissue, and reaction to shunt functioning. The effect of change of biomechanical properties of the brain might be greater than impact of a different valve used. The results of both studies revealed importance of individual analysis of intracranial dynamics in pediatric hydrocephalus before drainage system insertion and shunt optimization according to the type and opening valve pressure.

Location and adjacent tissue of the intraventricular end of ventricular catheter are an important prediction factor in relation to risk of shunt dysfunction. Location of ventricular catheter in the frontal and occipital horn of the lateral cerebral ventricle as well as a condition, in which the end of the catheter is surrounded by cerebrospinal fluid or touches the brain, can decrease risk of drainage system failure. Therefore, adequate design of a drainage system and appropriate location of the ventricular catheter are necessary for good control of size of the cerebral ventricles [318].

The analysis of sonographic morphometric parameters of the cerebral ventricles after successful drainage procedure in 40 neonates with hydrocephalus revealed a significant decrease of size of the cerebral ventricles. The drainage procedure had led to significant decrease of width of both lateral cerebral ventricles, bidirectional ventricular index, and width of the third cerebral ventricle. Before drainage procedure, progressive dilatation of the cerebral ventricles was observed in 36 (90%) cases and stable dilatation in 4 (10%) cases. During the early postsurgical stage after drainage procedure, regressive dilatation of the cerebral ventricles was observed in 31 (77.5%) cases and stable dilatation in 9 (22.5%) cases. Although drainage procedure (with increased ICP value measured before the surgery) had been performed, stable dilatation of the cerebral ventricles was observed in 10% of neonates with hydrocephalus. After drainage procedure, the clinical signs of intracranial hypertension had disappeared in the early postsurgical period. However, in 22.5% of cases, stable dilatation of the cerebral ventricles had been present after the surgery [319]. Also, other studies on pediatric hydrocephalus [28, 320, 321] confirmed decrease of size of the cerebral ventricles due to cerebrospinal fluid derivation when it was assessed by ultrasonography.

It is generally known that the use of CT examination is limited in suspicion of dysfunction of drainage system in children with hydrocephalus. It may be helpful to compare current CT image with the previous one when assessing dynamics of the intracranial lesion or size of CSF pathways. The previous CT images cannot be often accessed (entering the archive in the night, performing CT examination in a different hospital), which decreases validity of the examination. When CT examination shows progression of dilatation of the cerebral ventricles, it is usually a sign of blockage of drainage system. On the contrary, the stabilized size of the cerebral ventricles doesn't exclude acute blockage of the drainage system, in which an urgent neurosurgical intervention is needed [232]. Studies of various researchers refer to occurrence of dysfunction of drainage systems without change of size of the cerebral ventricles found in the CT image [227, 228, 322, 323].

The degree of dilatation of the cerebral ventricles depends on viscoelastic properties of the wall of the brain tissue [207]. Firstly, dilatation develops in the lateral cerebral ventricles. Then it spreads to the third cerebral ventricle, to the aqueduct, and finally to the fourth cerebral ventricle. This order is given by resistance of the brain tissue around the CSF pathways [324]. Slit ventricle syndrome may develop in children with chronic hyperdrainage of the cerebral ventricles [325–327]. In children with narrow cerebral ventricles, if obstruction of the shunt occurs, enlargement of the cerebral ventricles might not be seen in the CT image regardless of increased intracranial pressure [328]. Decreased re-expansibility of the cerebral ventricles can be caused by subependymal gliosis and decreased compliance of the wall of the cerebral ventricles and the brain tissue. At the same time, Laplace's law can play a role. According to it, to enlarge a compartment with low volume, greater pressure is necessary than for enlargement of a compartment of larger volume [224, 324, 329].

In cases of long-term inserted drainage system, changed biomechanical properties of the brain may be also responsible for different clinical manifestations of shunt dysfunction. In relation to drainage system obstruction, faster deterioration of neurological manifestations was observed in children with narrow lateral cerebral ventricles (Evans' index ≤ 0.35) than in children with large cerebral ventricles (Evans' index > 0.35). The predictive factors of decreased re-expansibility of the cerebral ventricles in shunt obstruction in children with hydrocephalus with indwelling drainage system are as follows: decreased size of the cerebral ventricles (Evans' index < 0.33), children over 3 years of age (if initial insertion of the shunt was performed in the first year of age), or period of 5 years after the first shunt insertion [330].

Nowadays, *ventriculostomy of the third cerebral ventricle* plays a significant role in the treatment of pediatric hydrocephalus. However, the long-term changes in intracranial dynamics after successful ETV have not been clearly described [215, 217, 318, 331–333]. The definition of successful ventriculostomy of the third cerebral ventricle also includes radiological criteria, emphasizing the clinical criteria [334]. Some studies revealed that successful performance of ETV did not decrease size of the cerebral ventricles [335, 336]. Results of the studies indicate that decrease of intracranial pressure does not have to be accompanied by change of size of the cerebral ventricles.

George et al. [337] studied changes of volume of the cerebral ventricles in children with hydrocephalus after successful performance of ETV. During longitudinal observation (24 months after surgery), they assessed volume of the cerebral ventricles as well as dynamics of the cerebral ventricles. If presurgical volume of the cerebral ventricles was greater than fivefold of the normal value, statistically significant decrease of volume of the cerebral ventricles appeared 3 up to 6 months after ETV. Even later the volume of the cerebral ventricles was the same. In the group of children with medium volume of the cerebral ventricles, which was measured before the surgery (less than fivefold of the normal value), less significant decrease of volume in the cerebral ventricles was observed 3–6 months after ETV. In the next period, volume of the cerebral ventricles was stable or slightly increased. In all cases, especially in the group of children with significant dilatation of the cerebral ventricles, volume of the cerebral ventricles after ETV was increased when compared to normal values. It can be caused by decreased absorption of cerebrospinal fluid. Based on the results mentioned above, the authors believe that successful ETV helps to create conditions for compensated communicating hydrocephalus. Impact of persistent dilatation of the cerebral ventricles on psychomotor development of a child is still the topic of the debate. Research of other authors confirmed that size of the cerebral ventricles did not change to the standard range after ETV [335, 338].

After successful ETV, clinical manifestations of intracranial hypertension can diminish in early postsurgical period. Despite the improvement of clinical condition of the child in the early postsurgical period, size of the cerebral ventricles did not change significantly [215, 335]. Indirect correlation between chronic hydrocephalus and decrease of size of the cerebral ventricles after ETV was observed. The longer hydrocephalus develops, the lower the decrease of volume of the cerebral ventricles after ETV was detected [336]. On the other hand, ETV does not always help to eliminate clinical manifestations of intracranial hypertension. Therefore, follow-up checkups of the cerebral ventricles may be helpful when assessing the effect of ETV [339].

Considering the type of drainage procedure applied (shunt or ETV) in children with chronic hydrocephalus, significant differences in effect on decrease of diameter of the head and size of the cerebral ventricles in postsurgical period were found. Decrease of diameter of the head and size of the cerebral ventricles in neonates and infants with obstructive hydrocephalus was more significant after shunt insertion than after the use of ETV [340].

In daily clinical practice, it may be difficult to perform visual assessment of change of volume of the cerebral ventricles, especially in cases with low decrease of volume of the cerebral ventricles and irregular-shaped cerebral ventricles [341]. Xenos et al. [316] found out that change of volume of the cerebral ventricles can be seen only if volume of the cerebral ventricles changed at least about 20%. Despite the fact that change of the cerebral ventricles is not visible 1 month after ETV, Schwarz et al. [342] found out that detailed measurement of parameters of the cerebral ventricles by CT can prove decrease of size of the third cerebral ventricle as well as both lateral cerebral ventricles.

In postsurgical period, successful ETV can change distribution of cerebrospinal fluid between the cerebral ventricles and subarachnoid space. Di Rocco et al. [343] confirmed progressive decrease of volume of the cerebral ventricles after ETV due to increase of liquor in the subarachnoid space. When stomy closed, distribution of cerebrospinal fluid regained properties typical for presurgical stage. Based on the results, assessment of change of CSF distribution between the cerebral ventricles and subarachnoid space is an appropriate indicator of ETV dysfunction.

Progressive dilatation of the cerebral ventricles occurred approximately in 25% of neonates with mild or moderate intraventricular hemorrhage and in 50–80% of neonates with the third stage of IVH and periventricular hemorrhagic brain infarction [28]. The stage of intraventricular hemorrhage in neonates can be diagnosed by the grading scale of Papile (**Table 12**) [344]. Recent data showed that only 15% of preterm neonates with severe intraventricular hemorrhage need permanent CSF drainage by drainage system [345]. Considering high morbidity and mortality,

1st degree	Isolated subependymal hemorrhage in germinal matrix
2nd degree	Hemorrhage in the lateral cerebral ventricle without dilatation
3rd degree	Hemorrhage in the lateral cerebral ventricle with acute dilatation
4th degree	Hemorrhage spread into the periventricular cerebral tissue

Table 12.
Classification of intracranial hemorrhage in neonates according to the scale of Papile [344].

management of *posthemorrhagic hydrocephalus* in preterm neonates with low birth weight is a topic of a great importance.

Drainage procedures in this age group are characterized by high risk of infectious and noninfectious conditions [346–348]. The list of drainage procedures includes repetitive lumbar puncture with CSF derivation (it is not preferred because of high risk of infections and insufficient amount of aspired CSF), external ventricular drainage, insertion of a subcutaneous reservoir followed by CSF derivation by repetitive aspirations, ventriculosubgaleal shunt, insertion of long-term internal drainage system (shunt), and endoscopic methods [349]. In relation to higher incidence of infectious and noninfectious conditions, subcutaneous reservoir insertion followed by intermittent aspiration of cerebrospinal fluid is applied more often than external ventricular drainage [350–352]. In preterm neonates with extremely low birth weight (<1000 g), implantation of subcutaneous reservoir is associated with high risk of complications [353].

Accurate value of volume of aspired cerebrospinal fluid and frequency of CSF derivation in neonates with posthemorrhagic hydrocephalus are often based on subjective assessment of clinical manifestations (degree of tension of the anterior fontanelle) and small changes of the cerebral ventricles detected by sonographic examination. In some extent, assessment of small changes of size of the cerebral ventricles by sonographic examination is subjective, and size of the cerebral ventricles does not often correlate with measured values of intracranial pressure [354].

Heep et al. [351] found out that volume of cerebrospinal fluid, which is necessary for prevention of progressive dilatation of the cerebral ventricles in cases with posthemorrhagic hydrocephalus, is not determined by child's weight but clinical manifestation. On the contrary, Bass et al. [202] performed direct continual measurement of intracranial pressure and found out that aspiration of 10 ml/kg volume of cerebrospinal fluid per day returns intracranial pressure to the normal values. In addition, they confirmed that regime of CSF derivation from subcutaneous reservoir leads to fluctuation of values of intracranial pressure. Volve (2001) also recommends volume of CSF derivation of 10–15 ml/kg per day in neonates with posthemorrhagic hydrocephalus.

Hunt et al. [355] analyzed the impact of derivation of cerebrospinal fluid on regional volume of the brain tissue in preterm neonates with progressive posthemorrhagic hydrocephalus. They performed volumetric examination by means of magnetic resonance. Derivation of sufficient volume of cerebrospinal fluid during puncture into the Rickham reservoir revealed increased volume of the gray matter about 39% and also increased volume of the myelin white matter about 61%. However, there was only minimum change in volume of demyelinated white matter and basal ganglia. Changes of the regional volumes after aspiration of cerebrospinal fluid provide new perspective on development of the brain in preterm neonates due to progressive posthemorrhagic dilatation of the cerebral ventricles.

Experimental studies on hydrocephalus confirmed morphological and biochemical changes in the cerebral cortex including impaired synaptogenesis and neuronal degeneration [356, 357]. Dilatation of the cerebral ventricles in progressive posthemorrhagic hydrocephalus has negative impact on differentiation of neurons in the gray matter due to axonal destruction [358]. Development of neuronal fibers plays a crucial role in development of cerebral gyrification [359]. Decrease of volume of the gray matter may provide an explanation for neurocognitive disorders in preterm neonates with posthemorrhagic hydrocephalus [360]. Based on confirmation of significant increase of volume of the gray matter in preterm neonates with posthemorrhagic hydrocephalus after derivation of cerebrospinal fluid, it can be assumed that early ventricular drainage has positive effect on psychomotor development of the child [315]. Besides the amount of extra- and intracranial factors resulting from child's immaturity, the final neurological condition is influenced also by the degree of intracranial hemorrhage and degree of destruction of the brain tissue [361, 362].

Even though neurosurgical procedures are usually performed after birth, *prenatal assessment of ventriculomegaly* is very important for prognosis of child's development, early termination of pregnancy, or early postnatal management of the child [363]. Ultrasonography plays a key role in investigation of ventriculomegaly in prenatal screening (**Figure 49**). In case of doubts in diagnosis or need of detailed assessment of the brain including the structures of the posterior cerebral fissure, fetal MRI examination can be performed. However, screening of the neural tube caudal defects by fetal MRI is not more effective than prenatal ultrasonography [365]. Ventriculomegaly is the most common developmental anomaly of the brain, which can occur during fetal period, approximately in 1 case per 1000 live-born children [366, 367]. Child's prognosis is mainly determined by occurrence of associated intra- and extracranial anomalies (2/3 of cases) and aneuploid lesions (9% of cases) [108, 368].

The term *isolated ventriculomegaly* describes dilation of the cerebral ventricles (width, diameter of the lateral cerebral ventricle in the level of glomus *plexus choroideus* >10 mm) without the presence of another developmental anomaly. The lateral cerebral ventricle in mild ventriculomegaly is 11–14 mm wide but ≥15 mm wide in severe ventriculomegaly.

Prognosis for development of the child, who is diagnosed ventriculomegaly by prenatal screening, is influenced by several factors:

1. *Width of the lateral cerebral ventricles*—a prognostic factor is width of the lateral cerebral ventricles ≥12 mm measured during sonographic examination of ventriculomegaly [364, 369–372]. The other studies revealed that prognosis is better in children with mild ventriculomegaly than in children with severe ventriculomegaly [108, 373].

2. The presence of *bilateral asymmetric ventriculomegaly* characterized by difference between width of the right and left lateral cerebral ventricle >2 mm is considered to be a negative prognostic factor [374]. Many studies confirmed good prognosis for children with unilateral ventriculomegaly [375–377].

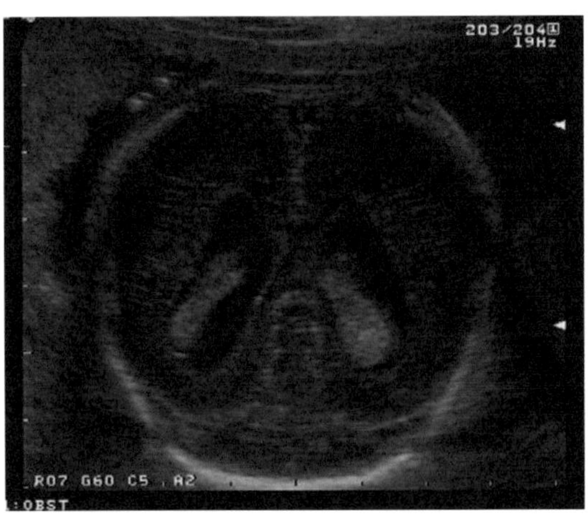

Figure 49.
Prenatal ultrasonographic screening of the brain of the fetus showing dilatation of the lateral cerebral ventricles [364].

3. *Dynamics of ventriculomegaly*—approximately in 85% of cases with isolated mild ventriculomegaly, size of the cerebral ventricles during intrauterine development returns to normal range of values, decreases, or stabilizes. Progression of size of the cerebral ventricles is a sign of unfavorable prognosis [364, 373].

4. During prenatal sonographic examination, not only width and asymmetry of the cerebral ventricles are measured but also morphological factors. It helps to predict *etiology of ventriculomegaly* and prognosis of the child, such as predilection sites of dilatation and shape of the cerebral ventricles, ependymal fissures, irregularity of walls of the cerebral ventricles, and destruction of the periventricular cerebral tissue [378].

14. Assessment of Doppler parameters of the cerebral arteries in children with hydrocephalus

Increased accumulation of cerebrospinal fluid in pediatric hydrocephalus leads to increased intracranial pressure, dilatation of the cerebral ventricles, decrease of intracranial compliance, and reduction of the brain tissue with negative impact on neurological condition of the child and his neurological development in the future. Alteration of cerebral circulation includes compression of the cerebral capillaries, stretching of the cerebral arteries, dysregulation of cerebral circulation, increase of cerebrospinal resistance, and decrease of cerebral blood flow. Progression of damage of the brain tissue results from decrease of cerebral blood flow and cerebral ischemia accompanied by changes in energetic metabolism (**Figure 17**). To measure reversibility of acute pathophysiological changes, and thus improve indication and timing of drainage procedure in a noninvasive way, there is a need for examination technique, which could be used in daily clinical practice. This is the potential of transcranial Doppler ultrasonography. It can analyze blood flow in the cerebral vessels and thus enables to perform noninvasive assessment of hemodynamic parameters of cerebral circulation.

Interpretation of changes in the Doppler curve of the cerebral arteries in pediatric hydrocephalus remains to be a discussed issue. Increase of cerebrovascular resistance of the cerebral arteries due to increased intracranial pressure is reflected in change of blood flow velocity and increased values of qualitative indices in the Doppler curve. Generally, there is good correlation between resistance index and pulsatility index of the cerebral arteries and intracranial pressure. Relationship between intracranial pressure, clinical manifestations of intracranial hypertension, dilatation of the cerebral ventricles, and Doppler parameters of the cerebral arteries is defined by biomechanical properties of the skull and the brain in various age groups. It may be also influenced by the amount of intra- and extracranial factors, which affect cerebral circulation [266, 289]. In critically ill children, several factors are usually combined, which may, but do not have to, affect changes in the Doppler curve of the cerebral arteries. Therefore, cerebral blood flow in this type of patients has to be assessed carefully [379].

Bada et al. [380] were the first who described *the relationship between Doppler parameters of cerebral circulation and intracranial pressure* in preterm neonates with posthemorrhagic hydrocephalus. The results showed increased resistance index of the cerebral arteries due to increased intracranial pressure. In the same year, Hill and Volpe [381] presented results of their research on changes of RI-ACA in neonates with hydrocephalus. In 9 out of 10 cases, dilatation of the cerebral ventricles was accompanied by increase of intracranial pressure. In all cases, RI-ACA was increased. It was affected mainly by decrease of Ved. But after drainage procedure, RI-ACA decreased due to increase of Ved. According to the authors, ventriculomegaly was considered a more significant factor influencing hemodynamic parameters of ACA than increased intracranial pressure. Because, in most of the cases, dilatation of the cerebral ventricles was accompanied by increased intracranial pressure, it is difficult to differentiate impact of dilatation of the cerebral ventricles from impact of increased intracranial pressure on cerebral circulation.

Fisher and Livingstone [382] observed change of parameters of blood flow in the Doppler curve of MCA, ACA, and ICA. The research revealed increase of PI, significant decrease of Ved, and slight decrease of Vsyst before drainage procedure. After drainage procedure, which is the functional internal drainage system, return of hemodynamic parameters to normal range of values was confirmed. However, this change was not accompanied by return of size of the cerebral ventricles to normal values, excluding width of the third cerebral ventricle. Correlation between size of the cerebral ventricles and Vsyst was not proven. Relationship between Ved and size of the cerebral ventricle was intraindividual in its nature. The strongest correlation was found between size of the cerebral ventricles and pulsatility index. Regarding morphological parameters, width of the third cerebral ventricle showed to be a precise indicator of changes of intracranial volume. It was found out that ACA and MCA have the highest predisposition to early reaction to change of intracranial dynamics [382, 383]. During observation of RI-ACA, RI-MCA, and RI-ICA in children with hydrocephalus before drainage procedure as well as in the early and later postsurgical periods, the biggest changes of blood flow Doppler parameters were found in the anterior cerebral artery [384]. In children with hydrocephalus, Nishimaki et al. [385] measured RI-ACA and RI-BA. They found out that both indices were significantly increased before drainage procedure, but RI-ACA was more increased than RI-BA. However, indices of both cerebral arteries were significantly increased after drainage procedure, and decrease of RI-ACA was more significant than RI-BA. Significant change of RI-ACA comparing with change of RI-BA before and after drainage procedure is probably determined by the anatomical location of the arteries. The anterior cerebral artery lies closely to the lateral cerebral ventricles, and the third cerebral ventricle and the basilar artery are located in the basal cistern in front of the pons. In most of the cases of hydrocephalus, the lateral cerebral ventricles are dilated more significantly than the third and the fourth cerebral ventricles. Therefore, the authors of the study assume that dilatation of cerebral ventricles has greater effect on the anterior cerebral arteries than on the basilar artery.

Although the basilar artery does not belong to the arteries with the highest predisposition to early reaction to volume-pressure changes in the intracranial space, assessment of increased RI-BA value and size of the cerebral ventricles, which had been performed in dogs with hydrocephalus, helped to distinguish cases, in which drainage procedure is necessary—with sensitivity of 77% and specificity of 94%. The value of neurological manifestations of symptomatic hydrocephalus correlated with RI-BA value and size of the cerebral ventricles. During measurement of individual dynamics, changes in clinical symptomatology had been accompanied by changes of RI-BA and size of the cerebral ventricles [386].

When observing changes of pulsatility index and cerebral artery resistance *in children with hydrocephalus before and after drainage procedure*, various studies revealed significant increase of PI and RI values of the cerebral arteries before drainage procedure and significant decrease of PI and RI in functional internal drainage system after surgery. Change of qualitative indices of the Doppler curve was affected by change of Ved. The results of studies showed that increased cerebrovascular resistance before drainage procedure was determined by increased intracranial pressure, which is reversible after drainage procedure. Positive impact of drainage procedure on Doppler parameters of the cerebral arteries is based on postsurgical change of cerebrovascular resistance and regulation of cerebral circulation due to decrease of intracranial pressure [319, 320, 384, 387–390].

The assessment of Doppler parameters of cerebral circulation and heart rate variability in preterm neonates with posthemorrhagic hydrocephalus showed that hemodynamic parameters as well as chronotropic regulation of cardiac function changed after drainage procedure [153]. A significant relationship between RI-MCA and PI-MCA was observed in the presurgical period in infants with congenital hydrocephalus [391].

On the contrary, van Bel et al. [392], who investigated 10 preterm neonates with posthemorrhagic hydrocephalus before drainage procedure, proved significant increase of PI-ACA resulting from significant increase of Vsyst. After successful drainage procedure, PI-ACA and Vsyst significantly decreased. The values of PI-ACA after drainage of cerebrospinal fluid were within standard range. When van Bel et al. [392] compared values of Ved and Vmean before and after drainage procedure, they did not find any significant changes. The authors of this study concluded that increase of PI-ACA before drainage procedure was determined only by increase of Vsyst. The same results were confirmed by Alvisi et al. [393]. Many researchers claim that increase of Vsyst before drainage procedure is caused by movement and compression of the anterior cerebral arteries through enlarged cerebral ventricles and flow of cerebrospinal fluid into the white matter, which results in decrease of transmural pressure gradient [393–395].

In neonates, infants, and older children, Goh et al. [396, 397] studied the relationship between intracranial pressure and resistance index of ACA and MCA. They found good intraindividual correlation between ICP and RI-ACA and RI-MCA in neonates and general good correlation between ICP and RI-ACA and RI-ACM in infants and older children. The difference between the age groups is probably caused by individual pressure-volume compensation of the intracranial pressure in neonates with hydrocephalus in various stages of hydrocephalus and various degrees of compliance of the skull and cranial sutures. Intracranial dynamics is more uniform in infants and older children. This corresponds with general good correlation between intracranial pressure and resistance index of the cerebral arteries. Significant decrease of RI-ACA and RI-MCA, determined by increase of Ved, was observed after drainage procedure in all age categories. Only in neonates, increase of Ved was accompanied by moderate increase of Vsyst and Vmean.

During continuous observation of blood flow in MCA by transcranial Doppler ultrasonography, positive impact of drainage of cerebrospinal fluid on Doppler parameters of MCA had been observed in children with hydrocephalus in the presurgical period while inserting ventriculoperitoneal shunt. Insertion of ventricular catheter into the lateral cerebral ventricle with CSF derivation led to obvious and immediate 30% increase of blood flow in MCA. When drainage procedure had been performed, values of PI-MCA, which were increased before the surgery, returned to standard range. The results of presurgical changes of Doppler parameters of MCA confirmed positive impact of CSF derivation on hemodynamic parameters of cerebral circulation in children with hydrocephalus [398].

Results of various studies emphasize the importance of data from assessment of changes of Doppler parameters of cerebral circulation to the record of *dilatation of cerebral ventricles*. Experiment on newborn rats with progressive communicating hydrocephalus showed that onset of dilatation of cerebral ventricles was not accompanied by alteration of parameters of the Doppler curve of the cerebral arteries. Pulsatility index of the cerebral arteries had been increased during development of hydrocephalus and followed by progression of ventricular dilatation.

This means that dilatation of cerebral ventricles did not change pulsatility index of the cerebral arteries. Instead, the change occurred due to progression of hydrocephalus and increase of intracranial pressure. It can be concluded that in this developmental stage of hydrocephalus, cerebral circulation was more influenced by increased intracranial pressure than by ventricular dilatation [399]. In chronic stage, changes of cerebral hemodynamics and advanced dilatation of cerebral ventricles were accompanied by other structural pathological changes [144].

Relation between *dynamics of dilatation of cerebral ventricles* (progressive, stable, or regressive) and basal and compressive values of RI-ACA was not found in neonates with hydrocephalus in the presurgical period. It means that dynamics of ventricular dilatation is not the only parameter influencing Doppler parameters of the cerebral arteries. In all cases of neonates with hydrocephalus, intracranial pressure was increased during drainage procedure, and clinical manifestations of intracranial hypertension had diminished after the surgery. Therefore, the authors of the study assume that Doppler parameters of the cerebral arteries are influenced by combination of increased intracranial pressure and dilatation of cerebral ventricles. Additionally, the results of the study confirmed that not only progressive but also stable dilatation of cerebral ventricles with increased intracranial pressure has a negative effect on cerebral circulation [319]. On the contrary, in neonates with stable dilatation of cerebral ventricles, in which drainage procedure was not necessary, basal Doppler parameters of blood flow in ACA reached normal values [400]. Similarly, Quinn and Pople [401] confirmed increase of PI-MCA in children with hydrocephalus who experienced dysfunction of drainage system. CT examination, however, revealed change of size of the lateral ventricles only in 10 out of 32 patients. Comparing with stable dilatation of cerebral ventricles, results showed increased value of PI-MCA and presence of clinical manifestations of dysfunction drainage system, in which surgical procedure is needed. When the procedure had been performed, PI-MCA significantly decreased. However, if intracranial pressure was not increased in stable dilatation of cerebral ventricles, resistance index of the cerebral arteries did not change either [402].

Not only increase of intracranial pressure and development of dilatation of cerebral ventricles but also changes of the cerebral arteries, such as distortion, compression, and stretching, may occur in pediatric hydrocephalus, especially in asymptomatic hydrocephalus [403].

The results of the study [319] targeted at children with hydrocephalus confirmed that *asymmetric dilatation of cerebral ventricles* had significantly influenced values of basal RI-ACA before drainage procedure and compressive RI-ACA after it. Statistical analysis showed that values of basal RI-ACA after drainage procedure and compressive RI-ACA before drainage procedure was not influenced by asymmetric dilatation of cerebral ventricles. Asymmetric dilatation of cerebral ventricles before drainage procedure may lead to stretching of the anterior cerebral arteries. When accompanied by increased intracranial pressure, it results in increase of cerebrovascular resistance and RI-ACA value. The presumption that asymmetry of the cerebral ventricles has significant impact on presurgical values of compressive RI-ACA was not confirmed. The authors of this study believe that it was caused by distribution of range of compressive RI-ACA before drainage procedure. In 36 neonates out of 40 (90%), compressive RI-ACA before drainage procedure reached maximal value of 1.0 regardless of asymmetric ventricular dilatation. In normal values of intracranial pressure after drainage procedure, the values of basal RI-ACA were not influenced by asymmetric dilatation of cerebral ventricles. In cases with standard values of intracranial pressure in asymmetric ventricular dilatation, dislocation of the anterior cerebral ventricles may occur without significant stretching and change of cerebrovascular resistance of anterior cerebral arteries. Compression of the anterior fontanelle in asymmetric ventricular dilatation, which is related to intracranial normotension, may worsen dislocation of the anterior cerebral ventricles if it is accompanied by increase of cerebrovascular resistance, resulting in values of compressive RI-ACA. Based on this study and clinical experience, the authors emphasize the fact that interpretation of Doppler parameters of the cerebral arteries in pediatric hydrocephalus with asymmetry of cerebral ventricles has to be done carefully [319].

In neonates with hydrocephalus, besides hydrocephalus itself, the following pathological changes of the periventricular cerebral tissue may also have negative impact on cerebral circulation: periventricular leukomalacia and peri- and intraventricular hemorrhage.

Impact of these changes on cerebral circulation and Doppler parameters of the cerebral arteries should be taken into consideration when assessing hemodynamic parameters of cerebral circulation in neonates with hydrocephalus in relation to observation of intracranial dynamics and indication of drainage procedure.

The most common cause of periventricular leukomalacia is perinatal infection (e.g., chorioamnionitis) and hypoxic-ischemic damage of the brain tissue. Considering various degrees of maturity of the brain tissue, consequences of hypoxic-ischemic brain injury differ in preterm neonates and in term neonates [28].

In preterm neonates, the periventricular white matter is at higher risk of hypoxia, which leads to focal or diffuse type of periventricular leukomalacia, while in term neonates, it is the white matter near the cerebral cortex, in which cortical and subcortical lesions of white matter can be detected [404].

The cystic leukomalacia lesions do not occur from the moment of insult of the brain tissue, but they develop continuously. At first, hyperechogenicity of the periventricular brain tissue is confirmed by a sonography. Then cystic lesions are formed during 10–14 days [405]. Pathological changes of structure of the periventricular brain tissue are accompanied by hemodynamic changes. Dysfunction of cerebral autoregulation was confirmed in preterm neonates with periventricular leukomalacia [27]. Many researchers also confirmed alteration of cerebral circulation in neonates with periventricular leukomalacia. By means of transcranial Doppler ultrasonography, Fukuda et al. [406] observed long-term decrease of blood flow velocity within all major cerebral arteries. In another research on periventricular leukomalacia in neonates with low birth weight, Fukuda et al. [407] confirmed that blood volume in ICA and VA had decreased a few days after birth and then between the 21st and 42nd day. Research by Ilves et al. [408] revealed that mean velocity of blood flow in ACA, MCA, ICA, and BA was increased in 83 asphystic term neonates due to severe hypoxic-ischemic encephalopathy during first days after asphyxia. However, increased mean blood flow velocity in the cerebral arteries was only short term. During the period of 21–59 days, it dropped below standard values of healthy term neonates. Changes of Doppler parameters of MCA in neonates with hypoxic-ischemic encephalopathy were also proven by Liu et al. [409]. In children with severe encephalopathy, the values of RI-MCA were <0.50 or RI-MCA >0.90 as a result of change of blood flow velocity in MCA.

To classify intracranial hemorrhage in neonates, the grading scale of Papile, which was created in 1978 (**Table 12**), is still being used [344]. In the past, it was assumed that grade IV denotes spread of subependymal bleeding into the surrounding brain tissue. Nowadays, decrease of venous drainage and development of venous hemorrhagic infarction are regarded to be the main triggers of intracerebral hemorrhage in neonates (Taylor, 1997) [28]. Subsequently, porencephalic cysts may develop in the site of periventricular venous infarction. In general, higher grades of intracranial hemorrhage lead to increased risk of severe neurological disorders in children. If grades III and IV of intracranial hemorrhage occur in active hydrocephalus, the brain tissue and cerebral circulation of a neonate are negatively affected by bleeding itself as well as changes related to increased intracranial pressure and progressive dilatation of cerebral ventricles. Moreover, there are many extracranial factors, which impact negatively on cerebral circulation, especially in preterm neonates [410–412]

Peri- and intracranial hemorrhage in neonates leads to dysfunction of regulation of cerebral circulation including autoregulation. Increased values of resistance index of the cerebral arteries, which were found out in the site of bleeding, are a sign of increased cerebrovascular resistance and presence of vasoconstriction near hemorrhagic lesions [264, 413]. Various research studies on neonates with posthemorrhagic hydrocephalus showed positive effect of drainage procedures and decrease of intracranial pressure on cerebral circulation.

The issue of frequency and appropriate time management of cerebrospinal fluid derivation during intermittent drainage in children with posthemorrhagic hydrocephalus remains open to debate. Large multicentric studies confirmed very low effect of frequent and early performed drainage, based on the assessment of size of the cerebral ventricles, in comparison with a conservative approach [414]. Since one of the prospective goals of intermittent drainage of cerebrospinal fluid is to prevent dysfunction of cerebral circulation due to increased intracranial pressure, changes of Doppler parameters of cerebral circulation in neonates with posthemorrhagic hydrocephalus have become a center of attention.

Nishimaki et al. [415] found out that values of RI-ACA in children with posthemorrhagic hydrocephalus were significantly increased before lumbar puncture or puncture of subcutaneous reservoir. But after aspiration of 5–10 ml/kg, they significantly decreased. Similarly, Kempley and Gamsu [416] confirmed decrease of intracranial pressure accompanied by significant increase of Vmean and decrease of PI-ACA, when CSF derivation had been performed in children with posthemorrhagic hydrocephalus. Quinn et al. [417] compared impact of increased intracranial pressure and CSF derivation on blood flow in ACA and internal cerebral vein (ICV) in neonates with posthemorrhagic hydrocephalus. RI-ACA was significantly increased before drainage procedure. But afterward, it decreased significantly. Changes of blood flow velocity in ACA weren't accompanied by change of blood flow velocity in ICV.

Maertzdorf et al. [418] observed hemodynamic parameters of ACA and MCA in the Doppler curve of preterm neonates with IVH and PHH during early gestation weeks. Aspirations of cerebrospinal fluid from subcutaneous reservoir of the ventricular catheter (type Ommaya) had been performed repetitively. When ICP before drainage procedure was ≥6 cm H_2O, then Ved and Vmean had increased significantly after performing aspiration. After derivation of CSF, when ICP was <6 cm H_2O, RI-ACA and RI-MCA had decreased. The value of Vsyst was not significantly changing after cerebrospinal fluid aspiration. The results confirmed good intraindividual correlation between RI-ACA, RI-MCA, and ICP in neonates with posthemorrhagic hydrocephalus. The use of infrared spectroscopy revealed that CSF derivation from subcutaneous reservoir leads not only to change of Doppler parameters of cerebral circulation, especially significant decrease of pulsatility index, but also to improvement of intravascular oxygenation of cerebral circulation [419, 420].

During assessment of effect of periventricular posthemorrhagic lesions on Doppler parameters of blood flow in ACA of neonates with hydrocephalus, significant correlation had been found between periventricular posthemorrhagic lesions and basal RI-ACA and compressive RI-ACA after drainage procedure. Before drainage procedure, Doppler parameters in ACA were influenced by increased intracranial pressure and also by posthemorrhagic lesions [319].

Based on the research, it can be concluded that derivation of cerebrospinal fluid in neonates with posthemorrhagic hydrocephalus leads to improvement of cerebral blood flow (**Figure 50**). While indicating and planning derivation of cerebrospinal fluid, changes of Doppler parameters of cerebral circulation should be taken into account [289, 421].

Doppler ultrasonography enables *assessment of hemodynamic parameters of cerebral circulation* of a fetus during prenatal sonographic screening. Comparison of findings with referential values may detect changes of cerebral circulation in various pathological conditions including fetal hydrocephalus [422]. During examination, a sonographic probe should touch the body gently because strong pressure can significantly increase RI, PI, and Vsyst and decrease Ved in MCA. But the Valsalva maneuver by mother doesn't affect Doppler parameters of blood flow in MCA [423]. Regarding prognosis and child management, the role of Doppler parameters of cerebral circulation as a complementary measurement in prenatal screening in fetal ventriculomegaly remains questionable.

Zalel et al. [424] did not find any correlation between widths of the lateral cerebral ventricles and RI-MCA in fetuses with normal size of the cerebral ventricles nor in six cases of ventriculomegaly. In the case of unilateral or bilateral mild fetal ventriculomegaly, no changes of Doppler parameters of blood flow in MCA were found in comparison to severe stage of ventriculomegaly [425]. Mai et al. [426] presuppose that examination of blood flow in MCA by Doppler ultrasonography does not provide new information regarding diagnosis and prognosis of fetal ventriculomegaly.

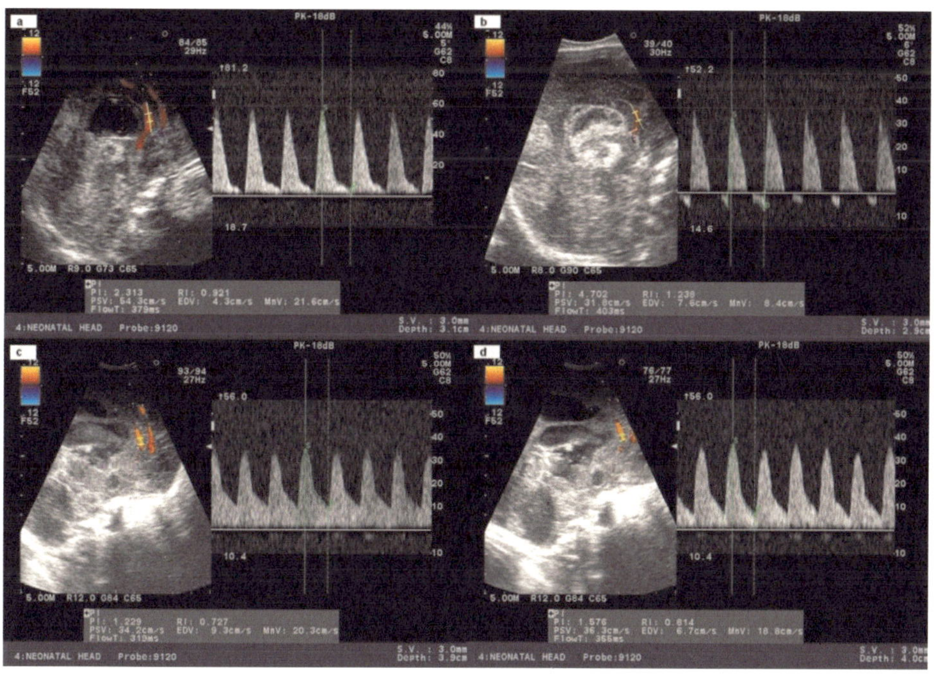

Figure 50.
Doppler parameters of blood flow in the anterior cerebral artery in the preterm neonate with posthemorrhagic hydrocephalus before and after drainage procedure. (a) Basal parameters before drainage procedure (increased RI, decreased Ved), (b) positive compressive test of the anterior fontanelle before drainage procedure (reverse blood flow during diastole), (c) basal parameters after drainage procedure (normal values of RI and Ved), (d) negative compressive test of the anterior fontanelle after drainage procedure; abbreviations used in the picture: RI, resistance index; EDV, end-diastolic velocity of blood flow; PSV, peak systolic velocity of blood flow; PI, pulsatility index; MnV, mean velocity of blood flow [319].

On the contrary, Voigt et al. [427] studied 143 cases of fetal hydrocephalus and confirmed that progressive dilatation of the cerebral ventricles results in increased cerebrovascular resistance and decreased cerebral blood flow. They concluded that assessment of changes of cerebral blood flow using Doppler ultrasonography helps to detect risk of brain tissue damage due to increased intracranial pressure and cerebral ischemia. To decrease secondary brain damage, drainage procedure should be performed early either in utero or postnatal after induced labor. Cavalheiro et al. [428, 429] confirmed that drainage procedure in utero between 24th and 32nd gestation week is of great importance in cases with isolated progressive infectious ventriculomegaly without signs of brain tissue destruction and chromosomal anomalies. Labor induction per C-section followed by postnatal drainage procedure is preferred from 32nd gestation week. Interdisciplinary collaboration, especially between a gynecologist, neonatologist, neurosurgeon, and anesthesiologist, is necessary when applying this procedure in clinical practice.

Changes of Doppler parameters of the cerebral arteries were found also in cases with *dysfunction of drainage system* after surgical revision.

Pople [430] focused on identification of referential values of PI-MCA in children with hydrocephalus with functional internal drainage system (**Table 13**). The sample included 248 asymptomatic children with hydrocephalus with functional shunt. They were 1 week to 16 years old. It is known that blood flow velocity in the cerebral arteries increases during aging. Changes of blood flow velocity in the cerebral arteries are more variable in children, especially in younger age groups, than in adults. The highest blood flow velocity was measured between the 3rd and 4th year of age. Since then it had been gradually decreasing to the level of values in adults. Pulsatility index had been significantly decreasing during the first 6 months of age. The lowest value was measured between 2nd and 6th year of age. Since then it had been gradually increasing up to the value of 0.9 in the age of 16. In addition to identification of referential values of PI-MCA in children with hydrocephalus with functional internal drainage system, Pople emphasized significant interindividual differences of Doppler parameters and importance of following the intraindividual trend [430]. In 63 children with hydrocephalus with dysfunction of drainage system, values of PI-MCA were compared with referential values. It was found out that

Age	Vsyst (cm/s) (mean)	Ved (cm/s) (mean)	Vmean (cm/s) (mean)	Pulsatility index (mean)	Number (n=248)
0–3 months	19–107 (63)	3–43 (23)	8–64 (36)	0.83–1.62 (1.23)	16
4–6 months	40–124 (82)	18–50 (34)	25–73 (49)	0.77–1.26 (1.01)	11
7–12 months	25–165 (95)	7–71 (39)	14–110 (62)	0.67–1.20 (0.94)	15
1–2 years	58–166 (112)	28–84 (56)	47–113 (75)	0.66–1.02 (0,82)	26
2–6 years	62–170 (116)	28–92 (60)	42–122 (82)	0.48–0.99 (0.74)	77
6–10 years	47–155 (101)	23–79 (51)	37–107 (67)	0.55–1.00 (0.77)	61
10–16 years	37–153 (95)	20–72 (56)	24–96 (60)	0.59–1.22 (0.89)	42

Table 13.
Referential values of PI-MCA in children with hydrocephalus with functional internal drainage system [430].

increase of PI-MCA determines shunt malfunction with sensitivity of 56% and specificity of 97%. The values of PI-MCA correlated with intracranial pressure of children with shunt obstruction [431]. Increased resistance index of the cerebral arteries was also confirmed in children with dysfunction of drainage systems [319, 320, 432].

In addition to increased resistance index of the cerebral arteries, vascular reactivity malfunction to p_aCO_2 change was detected in children with active hydrocephalus before drainage system insertion and in dysfunction of drainage system. When drainage system was inserted and dysfunctional shunt revised, resistance index decreased significantly. Then cerebrovascular reactivity to p_aCO_2 change had been improved, and that also led to functional cerebral circulation and regulation change [268].

Assessment of cerebral circulation by transcranial Doppler ultrasonography can be used not only to observed function of shunt but also ventriculostomy of the third cerebral ventricle. Vajda et al. [433] found out that PI-MCA significantly decreased in children with obstructive hydrocephalus after successful ETV. The difference was not statistically significant when they compared PI-MCA measured immediately after ETV with value measured in the 5th day after surgery. Effect of ventriculostomy was confirmed by assessment of cerebrospinal fluid flow using cine-phase MRI examination.

Clinical symptomatology improved immediately after the procedure in 17 out of 22 patients. Any correlation between PI-MCA and age or gender of children in the sample of patients was not found. The results showed importance of Doppler ultrasonography for observation of ETV function in the early postsurgical period.

Taylor et al. [270] used *compressive test on the anterior fontanelle* during TCCD examination in children with abnormal intracranial compliance. They studied basal values of RI-ACA and change of RI-ACA during the compressive test. The change was expressed as percentage difference in contrast to basal value. The basal values of RI-ACA of preterm neonates and neonates with abnormal intracranial compliance were significantly increased when compared to basal values of healthy term neonates. Only slight change of RI-MCA was observed in healthy preterm neonates and healthy term neonates during compression on the anterior fontanelle. However, RI-MCA was significantly increased in neonates with abnormal intracranial compliance. Basal values of RI-MCA were increased in neonates with increased intracranial pressure. Hemodynamic reaction of the cerebral arteries to compression of the anterior fontanelle had improved after drainage of cerebrospinal fluid. Compression test on the anterior fontanelle during TCCD examination can help to detect alteration of intracranial compliance before increase of intracranial pressure. The increase of ICP is manifested by increased basal values of RI. The study showed possibility of indirect noninvasive measurement of intracranial compliance and intracranial pressure by transcranial Doppler ultrasonography. In another study, Taylor et al. [269] assessed hemodynamic reaction of the anterior cerebral artery during compressive test on the anterior fontanelle in neonates with hydrocephalus. It revealed a significant increase of RI-ACA in neonates who were indicated for drainage procedure and in which increased intracranial pressure was confirmed by direct measurement.

Westra et al. [271] also dealt with the use of compressive test on the anterior fontanelle in children with hydrocephalus. They confirmed significantly increased basal and also compressive values of RI-ACA in pediatric hydrocephalus with increased intracranial pressure. A significant decrease of basal and compressive values of RI-ACA was found out when drainage procedure had been performed. Based on the results, they defined the boundary value of 0.70 for basal RI-ACA and 0.90 for compressive RI-ACA.

Gera et al. [434] focused on assessment of Doppler parameters of the anterior cerebral artery in relation to drainage procedure indication and change of measured Doppler parameters after drainage procedure. In children indicated for drainage procedure, they found out significantly increased value of basal RI-ACA and RI-ACA during compressive test. But after drainage procedure, the value of basal RI-ACA and compressive RI-ACA significantly decreased.

Change of Doppler parameters indicates increase of intracranial compliance after drainage procedure. However, any correlation between ICP and RI-ACA (both basal and compressive) was not found. The researchers believe that it is caused by complexity of the relationship between ICP and RI and potential nonlinearity of the relationship. During observation of RI-ACA in children with hydrocephalus in relation to indication of drainage procedure, the following values of basal RI-ACA were found out: sensitivity of 72.5%, specificity of 80%, and diagnostic accuracy of 75%. Assessment of RI-ACA by compressive test on the anterior fontanelle showed sensitivity of 75%, specificity of 100%, and diagnostic accuracy of 83.3%. False negativity in assessment of basal and compressive RI-ACA was the same (25%). **Table 14** presents comparison of the role of assessment of hemodynamic parameters of the cerebral arteries by Doppler ultrasonography during compressive test in children with hydrocephalus and indication of drainage system.

The compressive test on the anterior fontanelle increases sensitivity and specificity of resistance index and pulsatility index in regard to indirect measurement of increased intracranial pressure and decreased intracranial compliance in children with hydrocephalus. On the other hand, results of the compressive test require more careful assessment of effect of intra- and extracranial factors on cerebral circulation because their influence on compressive values is more significant than effect on basal values. Pressure applied to the anterior fontanelle during compressive test is defined within the range 0–200 g/cm^2. The pressure can gradually increase when using an ophthalmodynamometer [270]. When using a sonographic probe, shape (linear or convex) and size of a probe and pressure, which will be created by a doctor, need to be taken into consideration. Therefore, if a child was indicated for sonographic examination, it should be performed by the same doctor and the same probe. Regarding indirect measurement of intracranial hypertension and intracranial compliance, false positivity of compressive test can be found in preterm neonates who require intensive care (instability of extracranial factors), in severe stages of intra- and periventricular hemorrhage and dilatation of cerebral ventricles. False negativity of compressive test can be caused by CSF leak, subcutaneous CSF fistula, or small size of the anterior fontanelle [266, 319, 436].

Although transcranial Doppler sonography has been used for more than 30 years to assess Doppler parameters of cerebral circulation, interpretation of parameters in the Doppler curve of the cerebral arteries, intracranial pressure, intracranial compliance, and cerebral hemodynamics in pediatric hydrocephalus remains to be an open topic. On the one side, results of various studies showed possibility of indirect noninvasive assessment of intracranial pressure and compliance by means of transcranial Doppler sonography. On the other hand, results showed limitations and

	Taylor [435] (%)	Westra et al. [271] (%)	Gera et al. [434] (%)
Sensitivity	45	81	75
Specificity	95	100	100

Table 14.
The role of assessment of hemodynamic parameters of the cerebral arteries by Doppler ultrasonography during compressive test in children with hydrocephalus and indication of drainage system.

difficulties when assessing Doppler parameters of cerebral circulation in children with hydrocephalus. When assessing relation between intracranial pressure, resistance index, and pulsatility index of the cerebral arteries, wide range of factors, which can change shape and properties of the Doppler curve, need to be taken into consideration. Behrens et al. [437] used a mathematical model of cerebrospinal fluid circulation, which confirmed that relation between ICP and PI-MCA is significantly influenced by vascular compliance, autoregulation, and arterial pressure. They believe that individual variability of these physiological parameters is responsible for inaccurate reference of ICP value. Similarly, Hanlo et al. [438] confirmed decreased resistance index and pulsatility index of the cerebral vessels measured in children with progressive hydrocephalus after drainage procedure. However, during longitudinal simultaneous ICP/TCCD monitoring, correlation between ICP, RI, and PI was very weak. Based on the results, which showed a wide range of referential Doppler parameters of cerebral circulation and impact of extracranial factors, authors of this study believe that pulsatility index and resistance index of the cerebral vessels do not help in assessment of intracranial dynamics in patients with increased intracranial pressure.

This inconsistency of results on assessment of relationship between RI and PI of the cerebral vessels and intracranial pressure has led to research of more accurate noninvasive parameters of intracranial pressure. Hanlo et al. [439] presented new Doppler index known as trans-systolic time. The results confirmed that trans-systolic time of the cerebral arteries in the Doppler curve is less influenced by other factors (e.g., heart rate) and is more accurate for comparison of ICP, RI, and PI changes. Also, Leliefeld et al. [440] confirmed significant correlation between trans-systolic time and ICP. Despite these positive results, assessments of trans-systolic time of the cerebral arteries are not used for noninvasive measurement of intracranial pressure. It might be caused by a lack of referential range in children population and lack of experience with use in clinical practice. In another study, Leliefeld et al. [441] dealt with the possibility to use MR examination of cerebral circulation for indirect measurement of intracranial pressure. They found out that standard values of blood flow velocity in the brain and low values in ADC map were referred to compensated hydrocephalus without a need of drainage procedure. They claim that noninvasive changes of cerebral circulation by MR examination enable to distinguish the cases of compensated pediatric hydrocephalus with normal intracranial pressure without a need of drainage procedure from the cases of gradually progressive hydrocephalus with a need of drainage surgery.

Galarza and Lazareff [442] focused on clinical validity of transcranial Doppler ultrasonography in children with various types of hydrocephalus. The study showed that values of PI-MCA and RI-MCA were significantly higher in progressive hydrocephalus with a need of drainage procedure. On the other hand, RI-MCA and PI-MCA were not increased, and blood flow velocity in MCA was not decreased in the cases with compensated hydrocephalus (also known as arrested hydrocephalus) and ventriculomegaly (or essential ventriculomegaly). The results showed importance of transcranial Doppler sonography for indication of drainage procedure in children with hydrocephalus. However, the authors emphasize the importance of individual and careful assessment of Doppler parameters of cerebral circulation regarding pediatric hydrocephalus in clinical practice.

Rodríguez-Nuñez et al. [443] confirmed the role of clinical manifestations of intracranial hypertension, radiological morphometric parameters of the brain (Evans' index), biochemical parameters of cerebrospinal fluid (level of hypoxanthine, xanthine, and urea acid), and Doppler parameters of the cerebral circulation during assessment of pediatric hydrocephalus and indication of drainage procedure.

15. Case reports

15.1 Assessment of intracranial dynamics in the preterm neonate with hydrocephalus before and after insertion of external ventricular drainage

The preterm neonate (33rd gestation week) suffering from idiopathic hydrops with development of progressive hydrocephalus of four ventricles (posthemorrhagic, postinfectious) was indicated for insertion of external ventricular drainage. The mechanical ventilation in the child was used. Extracranial factors such as anemia, bronchopneumonia, and hepatopathy were presented. The neonate was 36 weeks old when drainage procedure was performed. Signs of intracranial hypertension were not clear in clinical manifestation before EVD insertion. Total body hydrops and edema of soft tissues caused difficulties in physical examination of the head. Enlargement of the cranial sutures was present, and the anterior fontanelle was opened, quite tense when palpated. The diameter of the head was not increased; it was stable regarding dynamics. Progressive dilatation of the cerebral ventricles with roundness of the horns of the lateral cerebral ventricles was confirmed by sonography. It was a sign of activity of hydrocephalus. Alteration of basal and compressive parameters of the Doppler curve of blood flow in ACA was found by transcranial Doppler ultrasonography (**Figures 51** and **52**). Drainage procedure confirmed increased value of ICP +13 cm of CSF column by direct

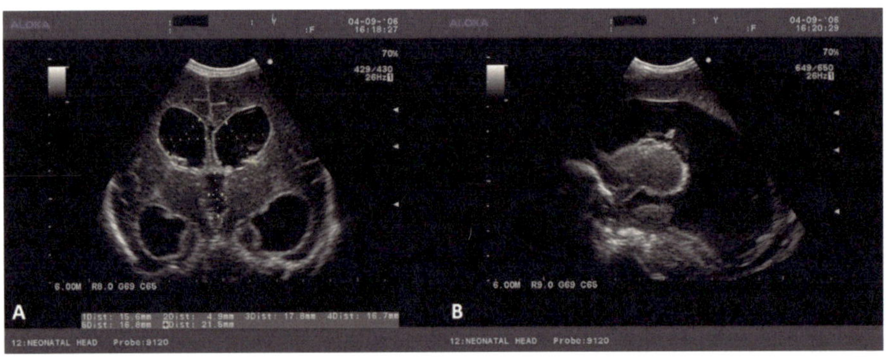

Figure 51.
Examination of the brain of the preterm neonate with hydrocephalus by transcranial Doppler ultrasonography before insertion of external ventricular drainage. (A) The coronal section, morphometry of the cerebral ventricles, (B) the sagittal section through the lateral cerebral ventricle. Roundness of the cerebral ventricles and significant dilatation in the trigonum. Occipital and frontal horns of the lateral cerebral ventricles can be seen.

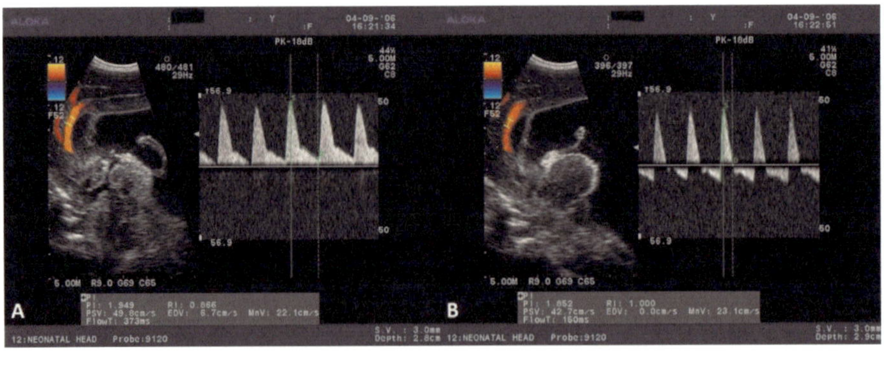

Figure 52.
The Doppler curve of blood flow in ACA of the preterm neonate with hydrocephalus before insertion of external ventricular drainage. (A) Basal parameters (decrease of Ved, increase of RI), (B) positive compressive test on the anterior fontanelle (reverse blood flow during diastole).

measurement. After insertion of external ventricular drainage, palpable finding on the anterior fontanelle (soft) changed, the diameter of the head decreased, and the distance between the cranial sutures diminished. Sonography showed significant decrease of size of the cerebral ventricles, which was accompanied by improvement of basal and compressive Doppler parameters of blood flow in ACA (**Figures 53** and **54**).

15.2 Observation of intraindividual dynamics in the preterm neonate with asphyxia and development of progressive hydrocephalus regarding indication of drainage procedure

The preterm neonate in 33rd gestation week. Immediately after birth, failure of respiration and the need of cardiopulmonary resuscitation were presented. In the first day after birth, ultrasonography of the brain revealed periventricular hyperechogenic lesions and moderate asymmetry of dilatation of the lateral cerebral ventricles with the asphyctic type of the Doppler curve of blood flow in ACA (low value of RI) (**Figure 55**).

The child was connected to mechanic ventilation. Slight increase of the head circumference, enlargement of the lambdoid suture, and tense anterior fontanelle

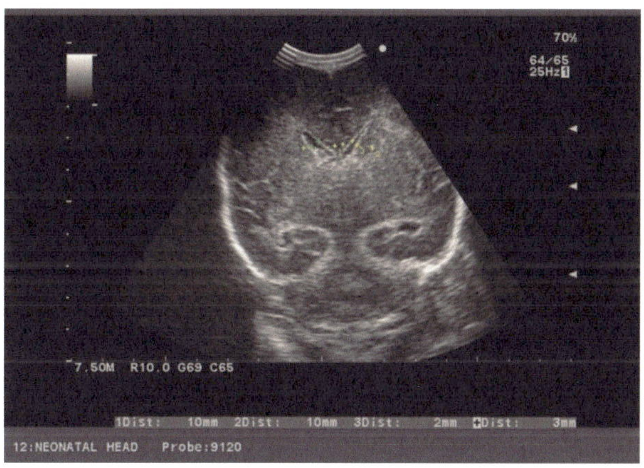

Figure 53.
Examination of the brain of the preterm neonate with hydrocephalus by transcranial Doppler ultrasonography after insertion of external ventricular drainage. The coronal section of the cerebral ventricles. Significant decrease of size of the lateral cerebral ventricles. The third cerebral ventricle is presented.

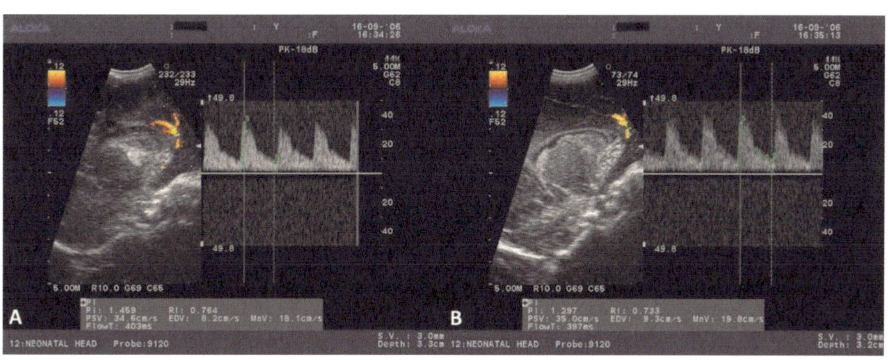

Figure 54.
The Doppler curve of blood flow in ACA of the preterm neonate with hydrocephalus after insertion of external ventricular drainage. (A) Basal parameters (postsurgical increase of Ved, decrease of RI), (B) negative compressive test on the anterior fontanelle.

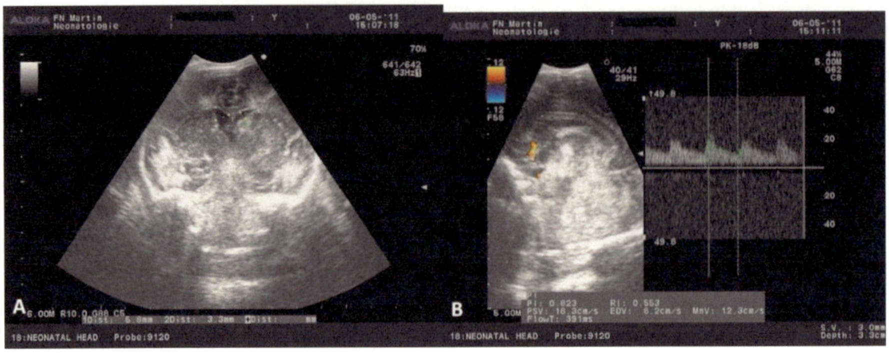

Figure 55.
Sonographic examination of the brain of the neonate with perinatal asphyxia, the first day after birth. (A) The coronal section, periventricular hyperechogenic lesion, moderate asymmetry of dilatation of the lateral cerebral ventricles, (B) the asphyctic type of the Doppler curve of blood flow in ACA, decreased RI.

were presented in the clinical picture. In the eighth day after birth, a checkup by sonographic examination of the brain confirmed progression of dilatation of the lateral cerebral ventricles and the third cerebral ventricle. Hemorrhage occurred in the third cerebral ventricle. Cystic periventricular leukomalacia had been developing when asphyxia had been eliminated. The change of the type of the Doppler curve of the blood flow in ACA was confirmed. The value of RI-ACA was in the normal range regarding age of the child. Compressive test on the anterior fontanelle was negative (**Figure 56**).

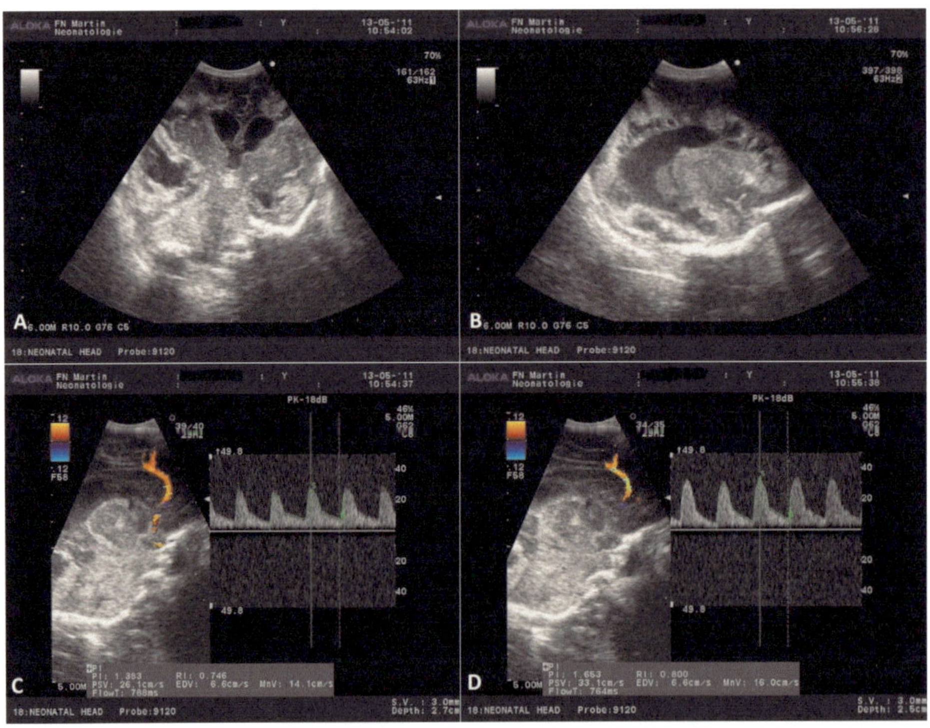

Figure 56.
Sonographic examination of the brain of the neonate with perinatal asphyxia, eighth day after birth. (A) The coronal section, progression of dilatation of the cerebral ventricles, hemorrhage in the third cerebral ventricle, development of cystic periventricular leukomalacia, (B) the sagittal section, development of cystic periventricular leukomalacia, dilatation of the lateral cerebral ventricles, (C) basal Doppler parameters of blood flow in ACA, basal RI-ACA within normal range, (D) compressive parameters of blood flow in ACA, negative compressive test.

Physical signs on the child's head changed 11 days after birth. Increased diameter of the head was accompanied by significant diastasis of the cranial sutures and tense anterior fontanelle when palpated. The child had been still connected to mechanical ventilation. Sonography showed progressive dilatation of the lateral cerebral ventricles, without change of the size of the third cerebral ventricle. Doppler parameters of blood flow in ACA had changed—basal value of RI-ACA was slightly increased, and compressive test on the frontal fontanelle was positive with end-diastolic block of blood flow (**Figure 57**). Regarding dynamics in the clinical manifestations of intracranial hypertension and sonographic image, ventricular puncture was performed. The value of directly measured ICP was 16 cm of CSF column. After derivation of 34 ml of cerebrospinal fluid, ICP decreased to the value of 6 cm of CSF column.

Ventricular puncture with cerebrospinal fluid derivation had led to short-term stabilization of intracranial hypertension. However, signs of activity of hydrocephalus were found in clinical manifestations again (tense anterior fontanelle, without bulging, diastasis of lambdoid suture, and increased head circumference). By means of one-time cerebrospinal fluid derivation, extracranial factors of the child had been stabilized for 10 days. Then, 21 days after birth, sonographic examination of the brain confirmed progression of dilatation of the lateral cerebral ventricles, communication of the right lateral cerebral ventricle, and cystic periventricular leukomalacia. The value of basal RI-ACA was slightly increased. While the anterior fontanelle had been compressed, reverse blood flow in ACA was presented

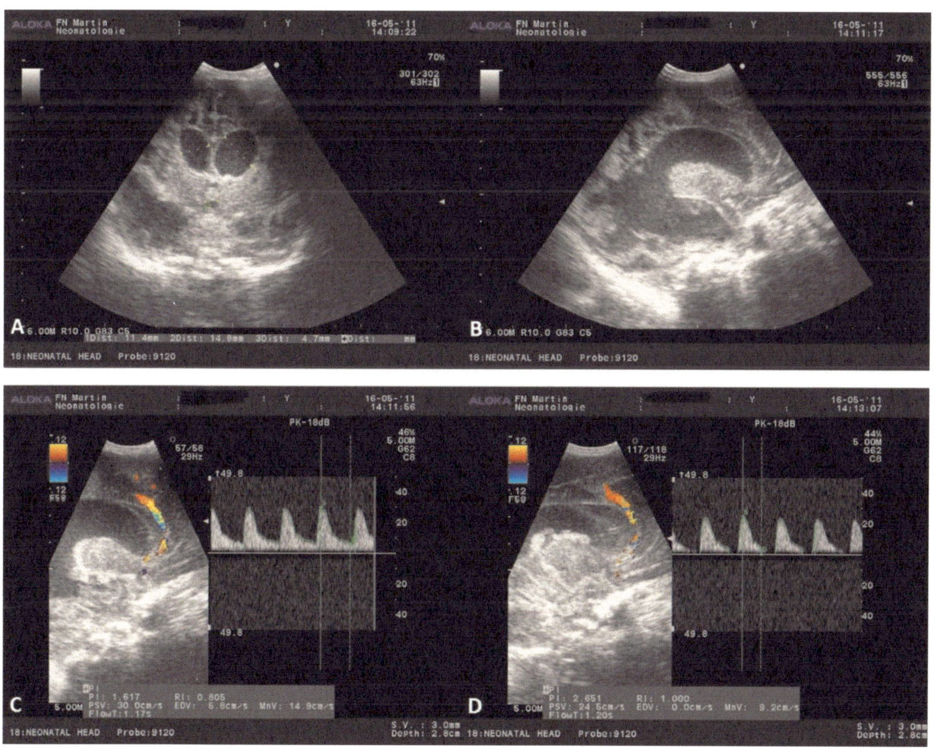

Figure 57.
Sonographic examination of the brain of the neonate with perinatal asphyxia, 11th day after birth. (A) The coronal section, progression of dilatation of the lateral cerebral ventricles with roundness of the frontal horns, (B) the sagittal section, progression of dilatation of the lateral cerebral ventricle in the trigonum and occipital horn, (C) basal parameters of blood flow in ACA, slightly increased value of RI-ACA, (D) positive compressive test on the anterior fontanelle, presence of end-diastolic block of blood flow in ACA.

(**Figure 58**). When assessment of dynamics of clinical and sonographic image had been done, the insertion of ventriculoperitoneal shunt was indicated.

15.3 Impact of tachycardia on Doppler parameters of blood flow in ACA in the infant with active hydrocephalus

Polystigmatized infant with hydrocephalus presenting with multiple congenital developmental anomalies such as congenital four-ventricular hydrocephalus, agenesis of corpus callosum, cavum septi pellucidi, ductus arteriosus Botalli apertus (condition after clipping), duodenal atresia (postsurgical condition), Meckel diverticulum (postsurgical condition), hypospadia glandis, and hypoplasia of the 12th pair of ribs. The child was born prematurely in 32nd gestation week. In the age of 1 year, signs of intracranial hypertension appeared. The clinical picture indicated activity of four-ventricular hydrocephalus, which had been stabilized up to that time. In clinical manifestation, increased head circumference with progressive dynamics of growth, tense and bulged anterior fontanelle, sunset eyes syndrome, and somnolence were presented. Transcranial sonography confirmed dilatation of cerebral ventricles. Low quality of the sonographic image disabled precise assessment of morphology of the brain and intracranial space (**Figure 59**). However, CT of the brain showed significant dilatation of cerebral ventricles and all the developmental anomalies of CNS mentioned above in the text.

Transcranial Doppler ultrasonography did not show increased values of RI-ACA and PI-ACA, while impact of severe tachycardia on the shape of the Doppler curve

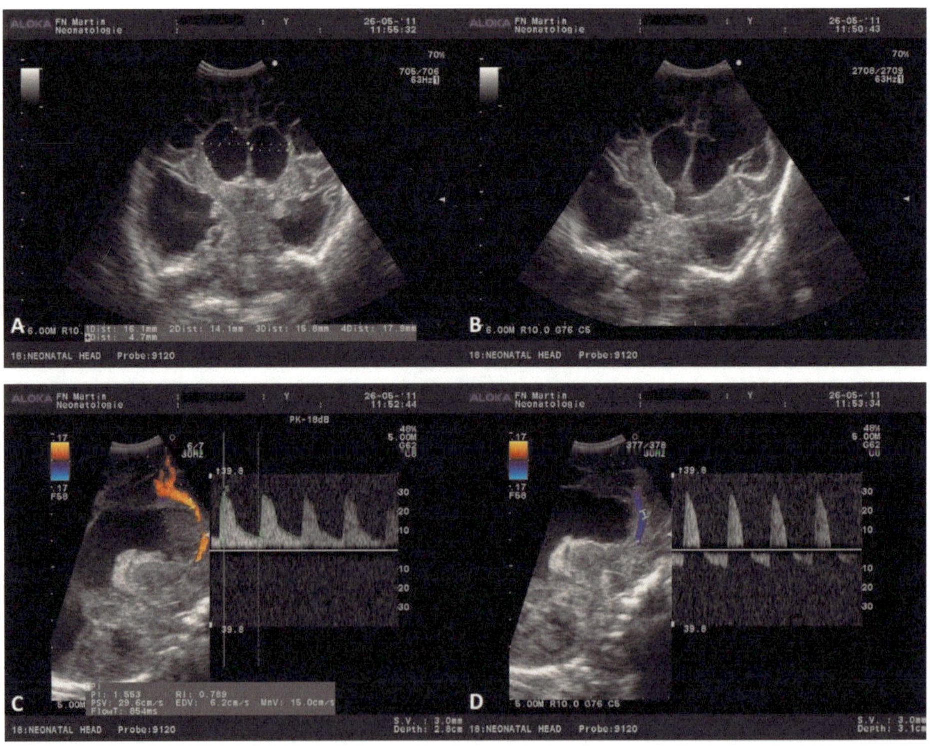

Figure 58.
Sonographic examination of the brain of the neonate with perinatal asphyxia and development of progressive hydrocephalus, 21st day after birth. (A) The coronal section, progression of dilatation of the lateral cerebral ventricles, stable width of the third cerebral ventricle, (B) the sagittal section, significant communication between the right lateral cerebral ventricle and cystic periventricular leukomalacia, (C) basal parameters of blood flow in ACA, slightly increased value of basal RI-ACA, (D) positive compressive test on the anterior fontanelle, presence of reverse blood flow in ACA during diastole.

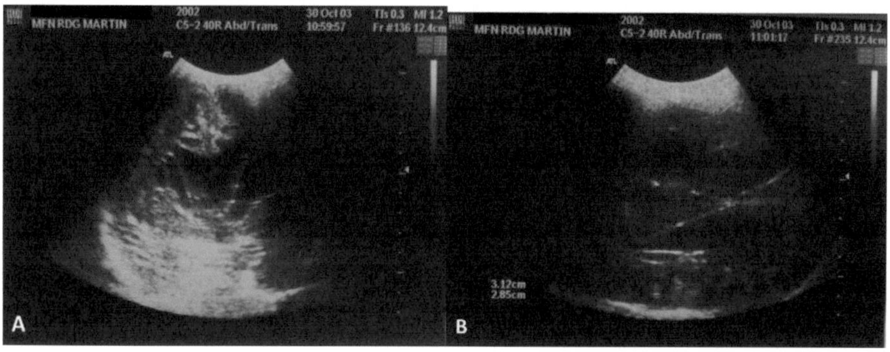

Figure 59.
The sonographic image of the brain of the infant with active four-ventricular hydrocephalus, agenesis corpus callosum and cavum septi pellucidi. The sonographic image is of low quality. (A) The coronal section, significant dilatation of the lateral cerebral ventricles and cavum septi pellucidi, (B) dilatation of both lateral cerebral ventricles.

of blood flow in ACA had been assessed by Doppler parameters. Considering signs of intracranial hypertension, insertion of ventriculoperitoneal shunt was indicated. Increased ICP value of CSF column of 14.5 cm was found out by direct measurement during surgery. The case study revealed a false-negative result of RI-ACA and PI-ACA assessment in regard to prediction of increased ICP in the infant with active hydrocephalus accompanied by tachycardia (**Figure 60**).

15.4 Assessment of intracranial dynamics of the infant with schizencephaly

In the child with schizencephaly, diagnosed by CT (**Figure 61**), clinical signs of intracranial hypertension (increased head circumference, tense and bulged anterior fontanelle, somnolence) appeared in the 11th month of age. Up to that time, the child was stabilized, dispensarized by the pediatric neurologist. Examination of blood flow in ACA by transcranial Doppler ultrasonography showed alteration of hemodynamic parameters of blood flow in ACA (decreased Ved, increased RI): Vsyst 84 cm/s, Ved 20 cm/s, and RI 0.76 (**Figure 62**). The ventriculoperitoneal shunt was inserted. After surgery, the child was more active, the anterior fontanelle

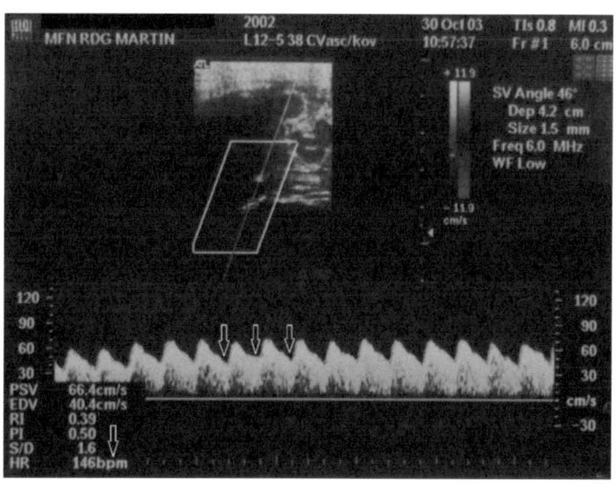

Figure 60.
The Doppler curve of blood flow in ACA of the infant with active hydrocephalus. Due to tachycardia, decreased values of RI-ACA and PI-ACA were measured, regardless of increased ICP value. The arrows point to cardiac frequency and diastolic segment of the Doppler curve (increased Ved due to tachycardia).

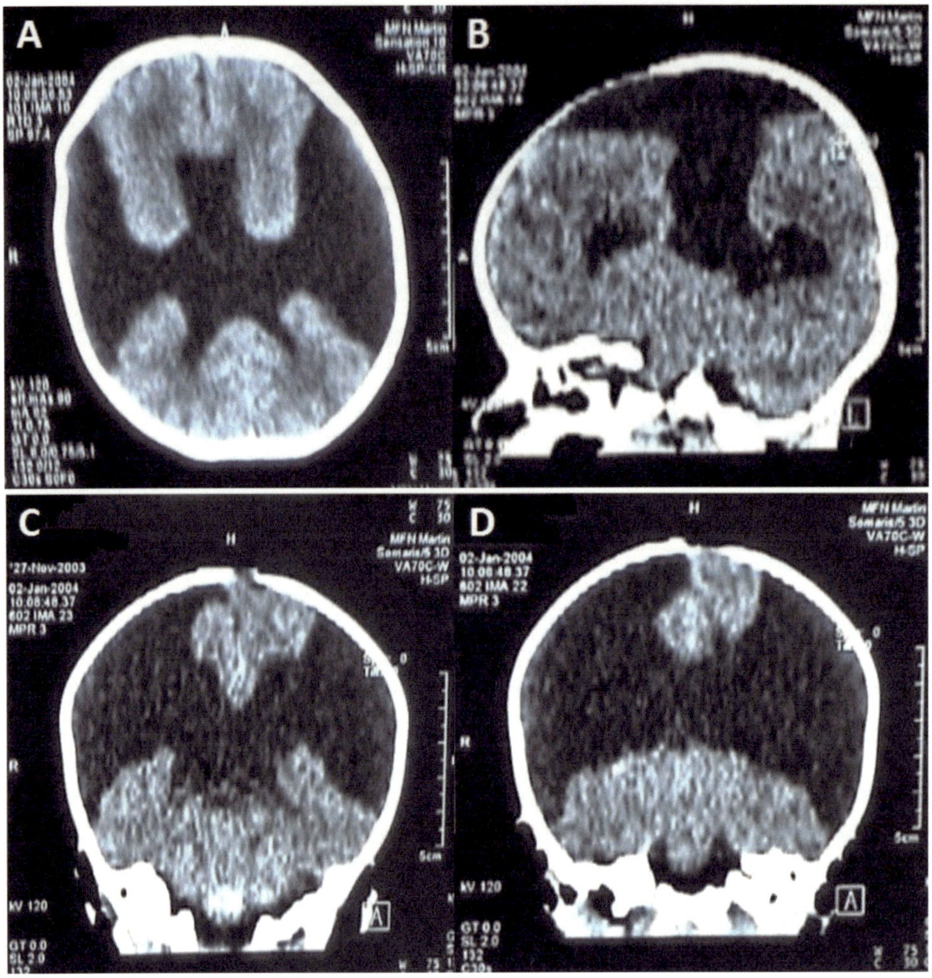

Figure 61.
CT examination of the infant with schizencephaly.

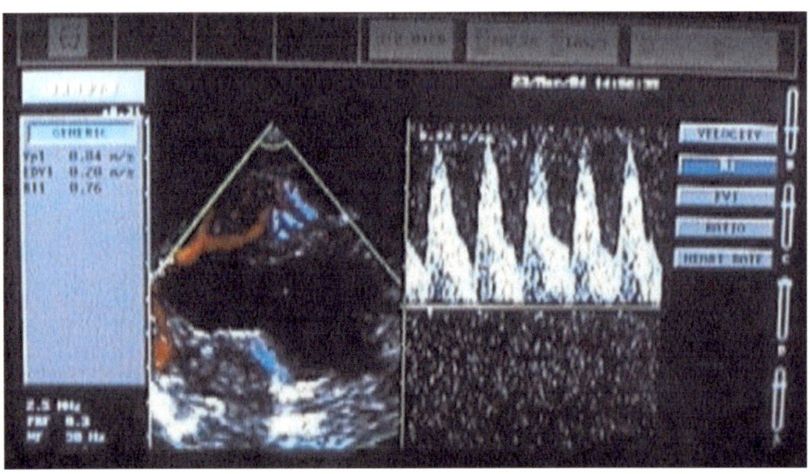

Figure 62.
The Doppler curve of blood flow in ACA of the infant with schizencephaly before ventriculoperitoneal shunt insertion. The value of RI-ACA is increased due to decrease of Ved.

was soft when palpated, and head circumference was stable. Also Doppler parameters of blood flow in ACA had improved when drainage procedure was performed (increased Ved, decreased RI): the basal parameters Vsyst 90 cm/s, Ved 34.8 cm/s, and RI 0.61; the compressive test on the anterior fontanelle was negative: Vsyst 85 cm/s, Ved 32 cm/s, and RI 0.613.

15.5 Assessment of intracranial dynamics in the term neonate with congenital hydrocephalus, Arnold-Chiari malformation type II, and lumbosacral myelomeningocele

The term neonate was born in 40th gestation week with open lumbosacral myelomeningocele. The neonate underwent the surgery up to 8 hours after birth closure of the caudal neural tube defect (**Figure 63**). Congenital hydrocephalus was detected by ultrasonography. Then MRI of the brain was performed. It revealed Arnold-Chiari malformation type II. Monitoring of intracranial dynamics was focused on the assessment of clinical picture and a sonographic image of the brain (USG, TCCD). The surgical wound was without CSF leak. The circumference of the head had been gradually increasing, the cranial sutures enlarged, and palpation examination on the anterior fontanelle changed (from soft it changed to tense fontanelle). No signs of deterioration were presented in the neurological status of the child. Checkup sonographic examination of the brain confirmed progressive dilatation of cerebral ventricles, which was accompanied by increase of basal RI-ACA and positive compressive test on the anterior fontanelle with end-diastolic blockage of blood flow (**Figure 64**). Ventriculoperitoneal shunt insertion was indicated because of the progression in the clinical and sonographic picture.

15.6 Assessment of intracranial dynamics in the preterm neonate with posthemorrhagic hydrocephalus

The preterm neonate was born in 28th gestation week. He was connected to mechanical ventilation after birth, blood circulation had to be supported by vasoconstrictors, and thrombocytopenia and bronchopulmonary dysplasia were presented. Hemorrhage into the germinal matrix and intraventricular hemorrhage with dilatation of the lateral cerebral ventricles (the third degree of the grading scale of Papile) was presented. No clinical signs of intracranial hypertension were presented in the child nor activity of posthemorrhagic hydrocephalus examined by transcranial sonography. Therefore the drainage procedure was not indicated.

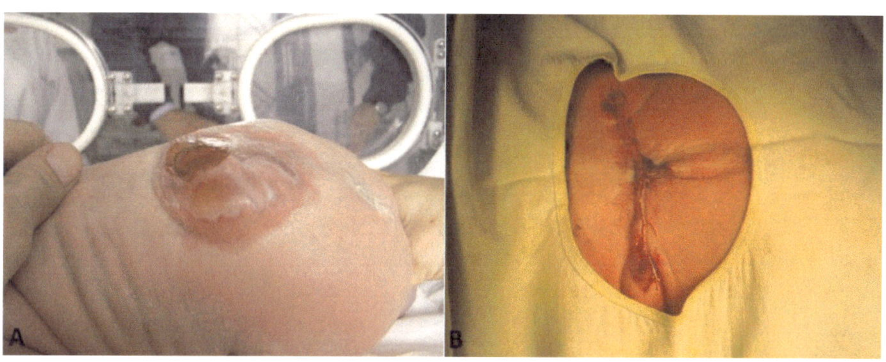

Figure 63.
The term neonate with Arnold-Chiari malformation type II, open lumbosacral myelomeningocele, and congenital hydrocephalus are presented. (A) The image of open lumbosacral myelomeningocele after birth, (B) the image of surgical wound after myelomeningocele closure.

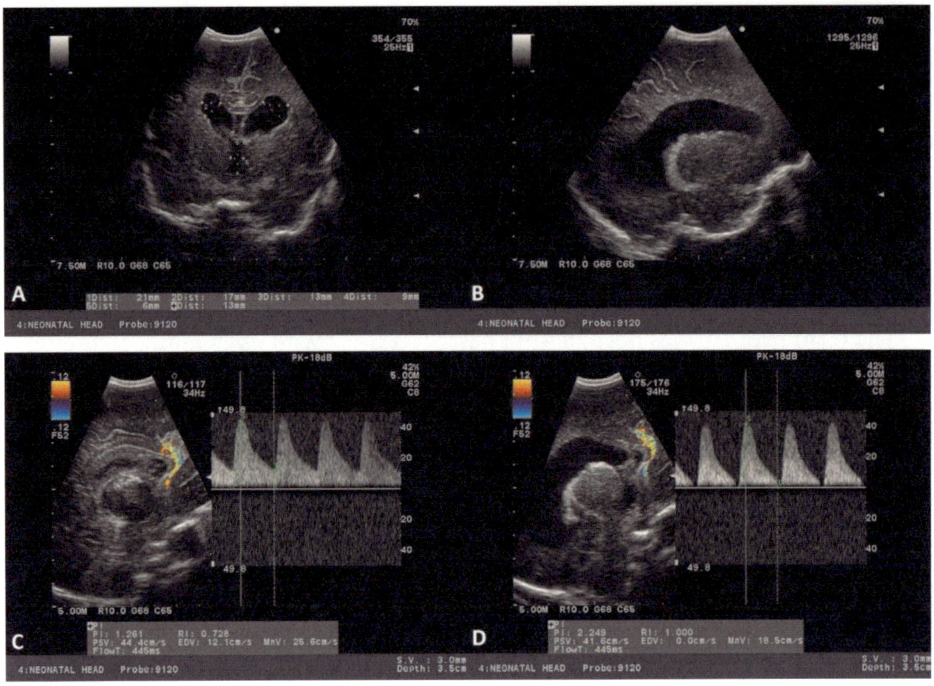

Figure 64.
Sonographic examination of the brain of the term neonate with Arnold-Chiari malformation type II and congenital hydrocephalus after surgical closure of lumbosacral myelomeningocele. (A) The sagittal section, dilatation of the lateral cerebral ventricles and the third cerebral ventricle, (B) the sagittal section, dilatation of the lateral cerebral ventricle, (C) the basal Doppler parameters of blood flow in ACA (increased RI, decreased Ved), (D) positive compressive test on the anterior fontanelle, end-diastolic blockage of blood flow.

Surgery for retinopathy and PDA was performed. Later clinical signs of intracranial hypertension had appeared, confirming the activity of hydrocephalus—diastasis of the cranial sutures, increase of head circumference, and tense anterior fontanelle. The child was connected to mechanical ventilation, and apathy combined with irritability of the child occurred. Sonographic examination showed progression of the dilatation of the lateral cerebral ventricles and the third cerebral ventricle with alteration of Doppler parameters of blood flow in ACA (**Figures 65** and **66**).

Puncture of the right lateral cerebral ventricle was performed. The value of directly measured ICP was of 15 cm of CSF column; after derivation of 14 ml of cerebrospinal fluid (sent to laboratory for biochemical and microbiological examination), ICP dropped to 5 ml of CSF column. After drainage procedure, it was found

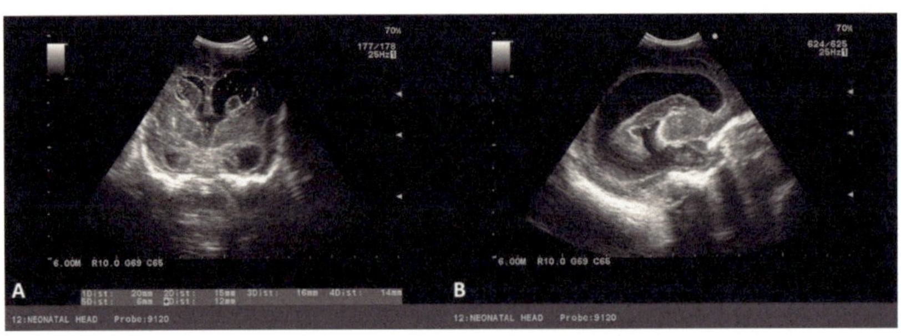

Figure 65.
Sonographic examination of the brain of the preterm neonate with posthemorrhagic hydrocephalus before ventricular puncture. (A) The coronal section, dilatation of the lateral cerebral ventricles and the third cerebral ventricle, intraventricular hemorrhage in both lateral cerebral ventricles and the third cerebral ventricle, (B) the sagittal section, dilatation of the right lateral cerebral ventricle.

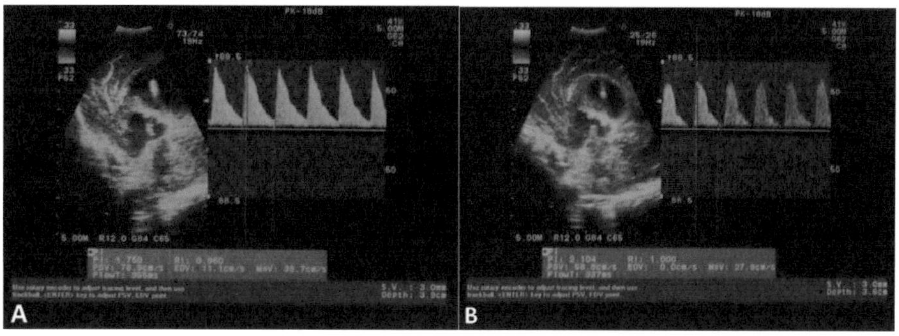

Figure 66.
The Doppler curve of blood flow in ACA of the preterm neonate with posthemorrhagic hydrocephalus before ventricular puncture. (A) The basal parameters, increased RI-ACA, decreased Ved, (B) positive compressive test on the anterior fontanelle, end-diastolic blockage of blood flow.

that the anterior fontanelle was soft when palpated. Derivation of sufficient amount of cerebrospinal fluid led to decrease of ICP to normal range accompanied by slight decrease of width of the lateral cerebral ventricles (width of the third cerebral ventricle remained the same) and improvement of Doppler parameters of blood flow in ACA (decreased RI-ACA and PI-ACA) (**Figures 67** and **68**). Overview of morphometric parameters of the cerebral ventricles and Doppler parameters of blood flow in ACA before and after cerebrospinal fluid derivation is presented in **Table 15**. Biochemical examination of cerebrospinal fluid confirmed increased concentration of proteins and increased amount of erythrocytes. Therefore, Rickham

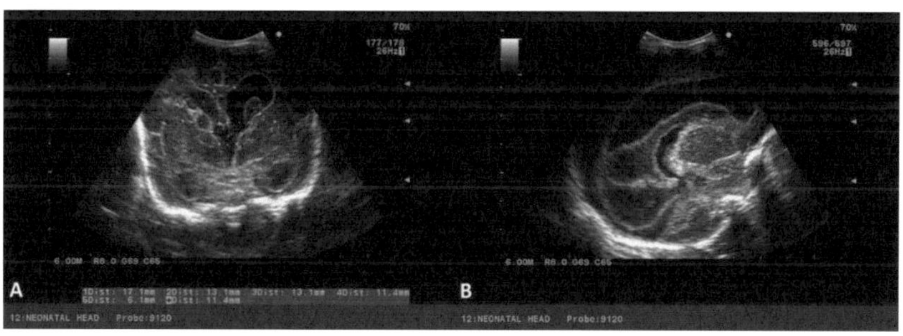

Figure 67.
Sonographic examination of the brain of the preterm neonate with posthemorrhagic hydrocephalus after ventricular puncture and cerebrospinal fluid derivation. (A) The coronal section, decreased width of the lateral cerebral ventricles, width of the third cerebral ventricle was the same, (B) the sagittal section, dilatation of the right lateral cerebral ventricle.

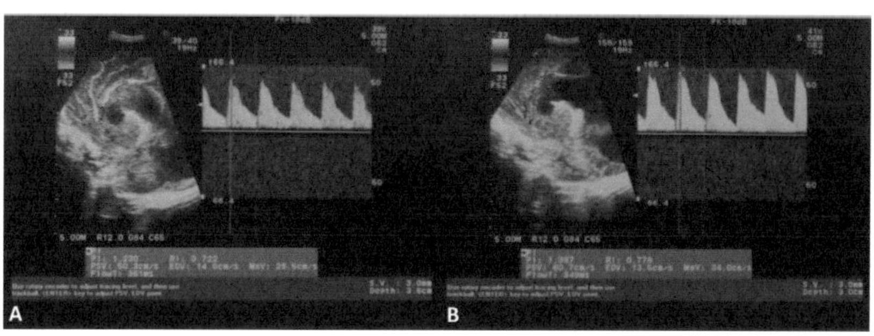

Figure 68.
The Doppler curve of blood flow in ACA of the preterm neonate with posthemorrhagic hydrocephalus after ventricular puncture and cerebrospinal fluid derivation. (A) Normal basal parameters, decrease of RI-ACA due to increase of Ved, (B) negative compressive test on the anterior fontanelle.

Parameters	Before CSF derivation	After CSF derivation
Morphometric parameters		
Width of right lateral cerebral ventricle (mm)	16	13.1
Width of left lateral cerebral ventricle (mm)	14	11.4
Ventricular index of right lateral cerebral ventricle (mm)	20	17.1
Ventricular index of left lateral cerebral ventricle (mm)	15	13.1
Width of the third cerebral ventricle (mm)	6	6.1
Basal Doppler parameters		
Vsyst (cm/s)	78.9	50.3
Ved (cm/s)	11.1	14.0
Vmean (cm/s)	38.7	29.5
Resistance index (RI)	0.860	0.722
Pulsatility index (PI)	1.750	1.230
Compressive Doppler parameters		
Vsyst (cm/s)	58.8	60.7
Ved (cm/s)	0	13.5
Vmean (cm/s)	27.9	34.0
Resistance index (RI)	1.00	0.778
Pulsatility index (PI)	2.104	1.387
ICP value (cm of CSF column)	15	5

Table 15.
Morphometric parameters of the cerebral ventricles and Doppler parameters of blood flow in ACA of the preterm neonate with posthemorrhagic hydrocephalus before and after ventricular puncture and cerebrospinal fluid derivation.

subcutaneous reservoir was inserted. Ventriculoperitoneal shunt insertion was performed after three-week-long period of cerebrospinal fluid derivations from reservoir.

15.7 Assessment of intracranial dynamics in the neonate with occipital encephalocele and congenital hydrocephalus

The term neonate was born in 23rd gestation week suffering from occipital encephalocele and congenital hydrocephalus (**Figure 69**). CT examination was performed in the day of birth. It showed three-ventricular obstructive hydrocephalus and occipital encephalocele. Dilatation of the lateral cerebral ventricles was dominant on the CT image (**Figures 70** and **71**). Examination of blood flow in ACA by transcranial Doppler ultrasonography confirmed alteration of basal parameters: increased RI-ACA (**Figure 72**).

The following signs of intracranial hypertension were found in clinical manifestation: widely enlarged and tense anterior fontanelle, diastasis of cranial sutures, and enlarged head circumference. Compression of the anterior fontanelle caused bradycardia. Occipital encephalocele resection and ventriculoperitoneal shunt insertion during one operation were performed.

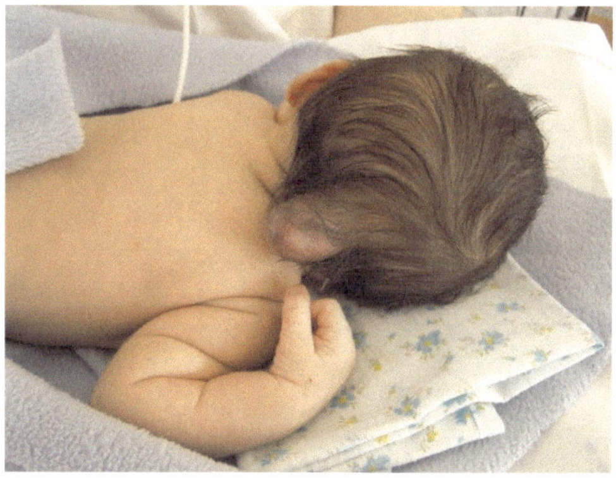

Figure 69.
The neonate with the occipital encephalocele.

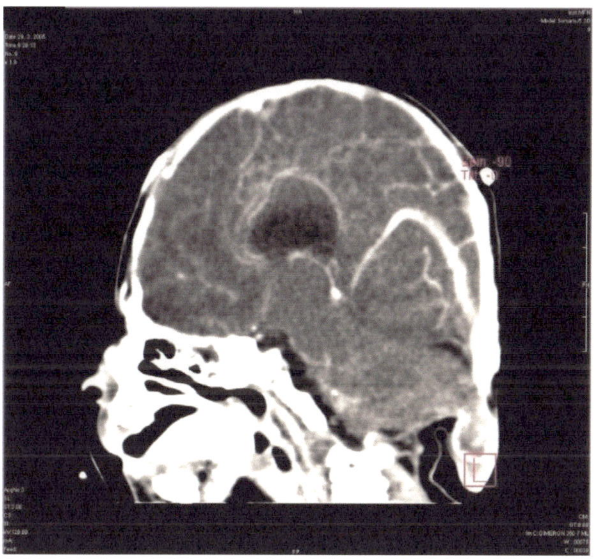

Figure 70.
CT examination of the brain of the neonate with occipital encephalocele (the sagittal section).

After surgery, the anterior fontanelle was soft when palpated, head circumference did not change in the early postoperative period, and diastasis of the sagittal suture and anterior fontanelle was presented. CT checkup examination was performed 14 days after surgery. It showed significant decrease of the size of right lateral cerebral ventricle, asymmetry width of the lateral cerebral ventricles, and movement of the septum pellucidum to the right by 4 mm (**Figure 73**).

The parameters of the Doppler curve in ACA were as follows: basal, Vsyst 48.3 cm/s, Ved 14 cm/s, and RI 0.711 (boundary value RI); compressive, Vsyst 55.3 cm/s, Ved 5.12 cm/s, and RI 0.91 (positive compressive test). The clinical signs of intracranial hypertension were not presented after surgery. Impact of asymmetry of the lateral cerebral ventricles and midline shift on Doppler parameters of blood flow in ACA might cause the alteration of Doppler parameters, especially during compressive test on the anterior fontanelle. The impact of asymmetry of the lateral cerebral ventricles on Doppler parameters of the anterior cerebral arteries was described in the study by Kolarovszki et al. [319].

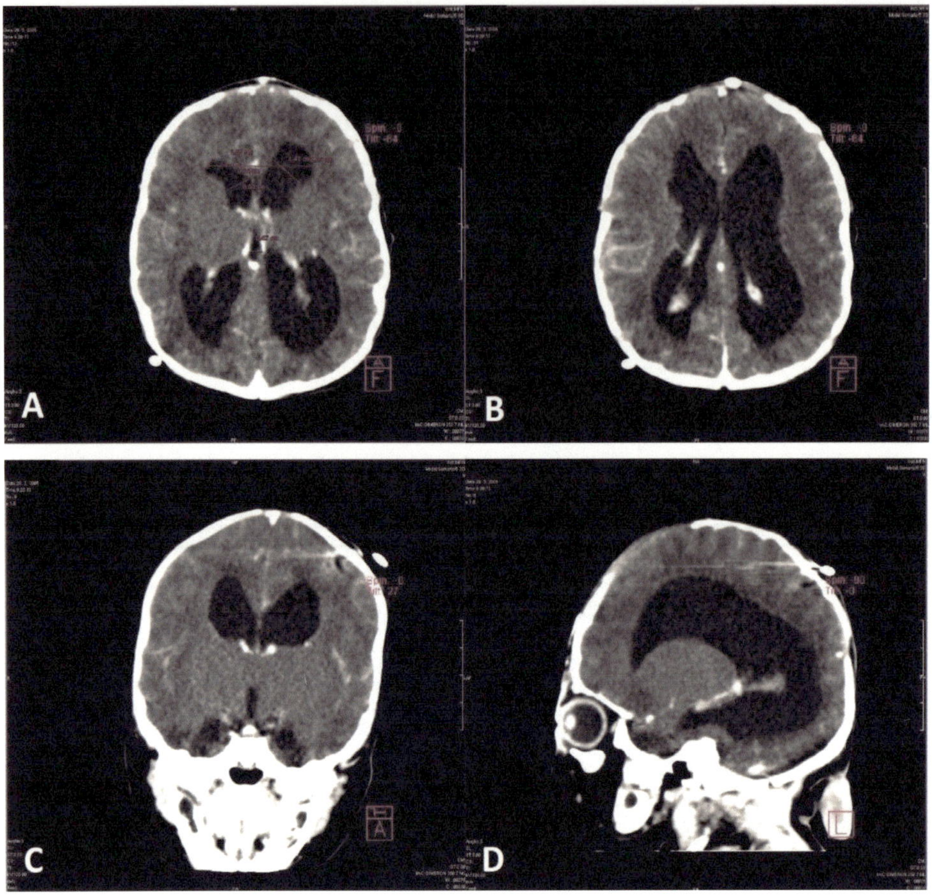

Figure 71.
CT examination of the neonate with congenital three-ventricular hydrocephalus and occipital encephalocele. Dilatation of the lateral cerebral ventricles. The third cerebral ventricle is enlarged in CT image.

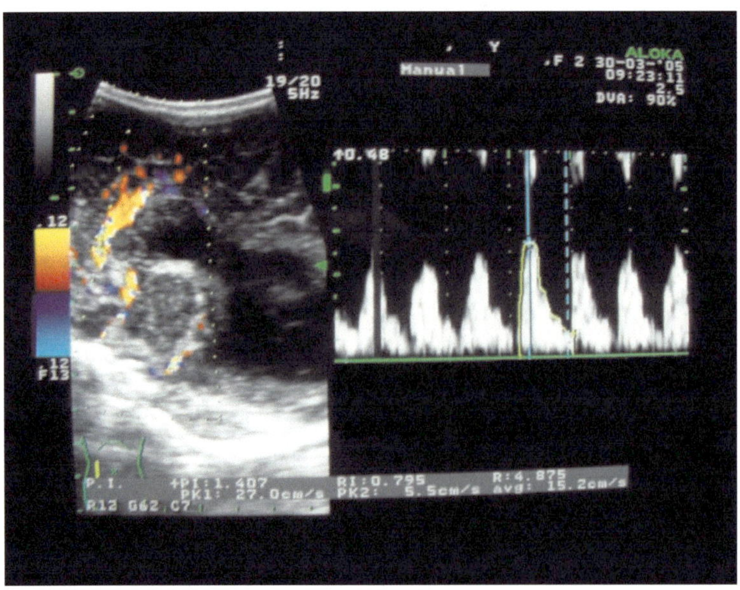

Figure 72.
The Doppler curve of blood flow in ACA of the neonate with congenital three-ventricular hydrocephalus and occipital encephalocele. Basal parameters—increased RI-ACA, decreased Ved.

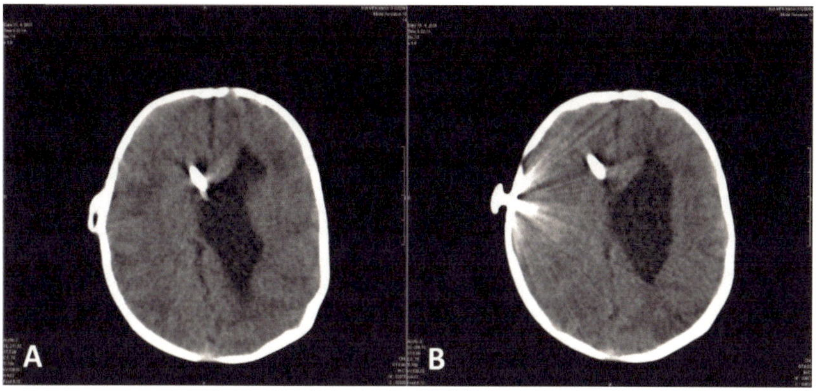

Figure 73.
CT of the brain (A, B–axial plane) of the neonate with congenital three-ventricular hydrocephalus after ventriculoperitoneal shunt insertion. Significant decrease of width of the right lateral cerebral ventricle, asymmetry of the lateral cerebral ventricles.

15.8 Assessment of intracranial dynamics in the term neonate with birth trauma, intracerebral hemorrhage, and hemocephalus

The term neonate born in 38th gestation week was in the first day after birth transported to the Clinic of Neonatology of the Jessenius Faculty of Medicine and the University Hospital Martin from a regional hospital. According to the medical record, the child was born by occiput. But instrumental labor was not mentioned in the medical record. On admission, blue mask syndrome (stagnation cyanosis of the face), large cephalhematoma, and swelling of soft tissues of the head were presented (**Figure 74**). Signs of intracranial hypertension were not presented. The frontal fontanelle was in niveau, soft when palpated, pupils were isocoric, and symmetric movement of the extremities was presented. The subclinical seizure activity was shown on the continual aEEG image.

Severe hemorrhage in right cerebral hemisphere and blood in the lateral cerebral ventricles and in the third cerebral ventricle were shown by sonography (**Figure 75**). Basal parameters of the Doppler curve in ACA were altered and Vsyst, Ved, and Vmean decreased. Regarding significant decrease of Ved, the value of RI was increased (**Figure 76**).

CT examination was done on the day of admission because of the finding in the sonographic image. It confirmed severe intracerebral hemorrhage (parieto-occipital right), which spread into the ventricular system, hemocephalus without development of acute obstructive hydrocephalus, subdural hematoma above the tentorium

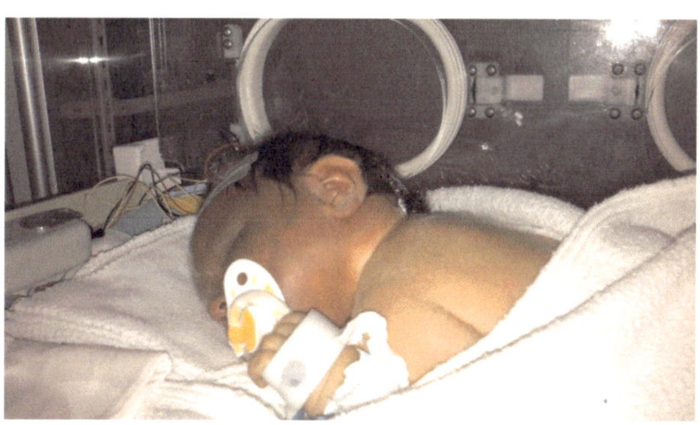

Figure 74.
The term neonate with blue mask syndrome. Stagnation cyanosis of the face. Continual aEEG monitoring.

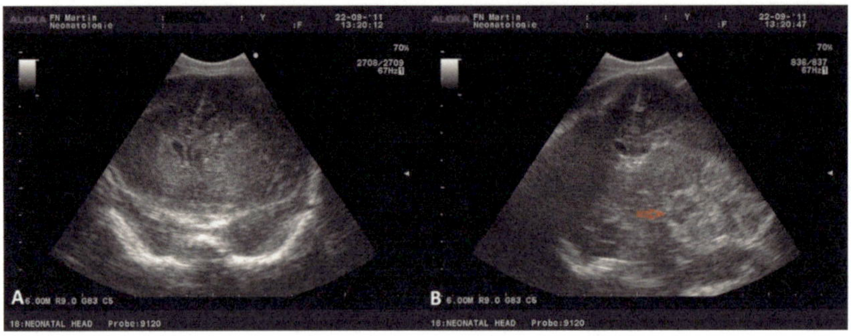

Figure 75.
Sonographic examination of the neonate after birth trauma, the first day after birth. (A) The sagittal section, significant shift of the septum pellucidum to the left, hemorrhage in both lateral cerebral ventricles and in the third cerebral ventricle and hemorrhage in the right cerebral hemisphere, (B) the coronal section, significant hemorrhage in both lateral cerebral ventricles and in the third cerebral ventricle and hemorrhage in the right cerebral hemisphere.

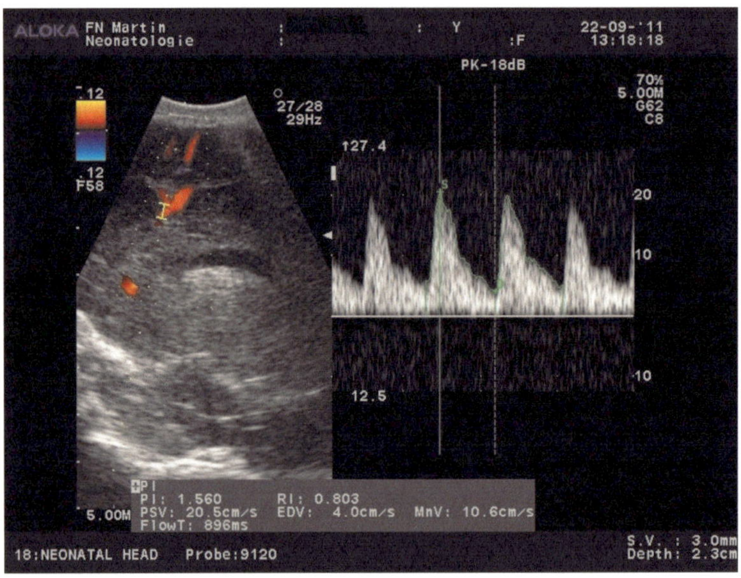

Figure 76.
The Doppler curve of the blood flow in ACA in the neonate after severe birth trauma, the first day after birth. Decreased blood flow velocity (↓Vsyst, ↓Ved, and ↓Vmean). Value of RI-ACA is significantly increased due to significant decrease of Ved.

on the right, and shift of the septum pellucidum by 7 mm to the left. Also, graphic image of cephalhematoma, swelling of the soft brain tissue, and impression of the occipital bone into the intracranial space around the lambdoid suture (**Figures 77** and **78**) were presented. Clinical finding on the head and result of CT examination pointed out the diagnosis of birth trauma. MRI of the brain did not show cerebral anomalies or brain tumor.

The second day after birth, the neonate's condition was stabilized, without signs of intracranial hypertension, subclinical spasm activity was shown by aEEG, and in neurological status the hyperreflexia was presented. Checkup sonography of the brain confirmed stable finding of intracranial hemorrhage, without development of obstructive hydrocephalus (**Figure 79**). For the increased blood flow velocity in ACA, value of RI-ACA was only slightly increased (**Figure 80**). Because of the risk of effect of the midline shift to Doppler parameters of blood flow in ACA, parameters of the Doppler curve of blood flow in BA were assessed as well. Blood flow

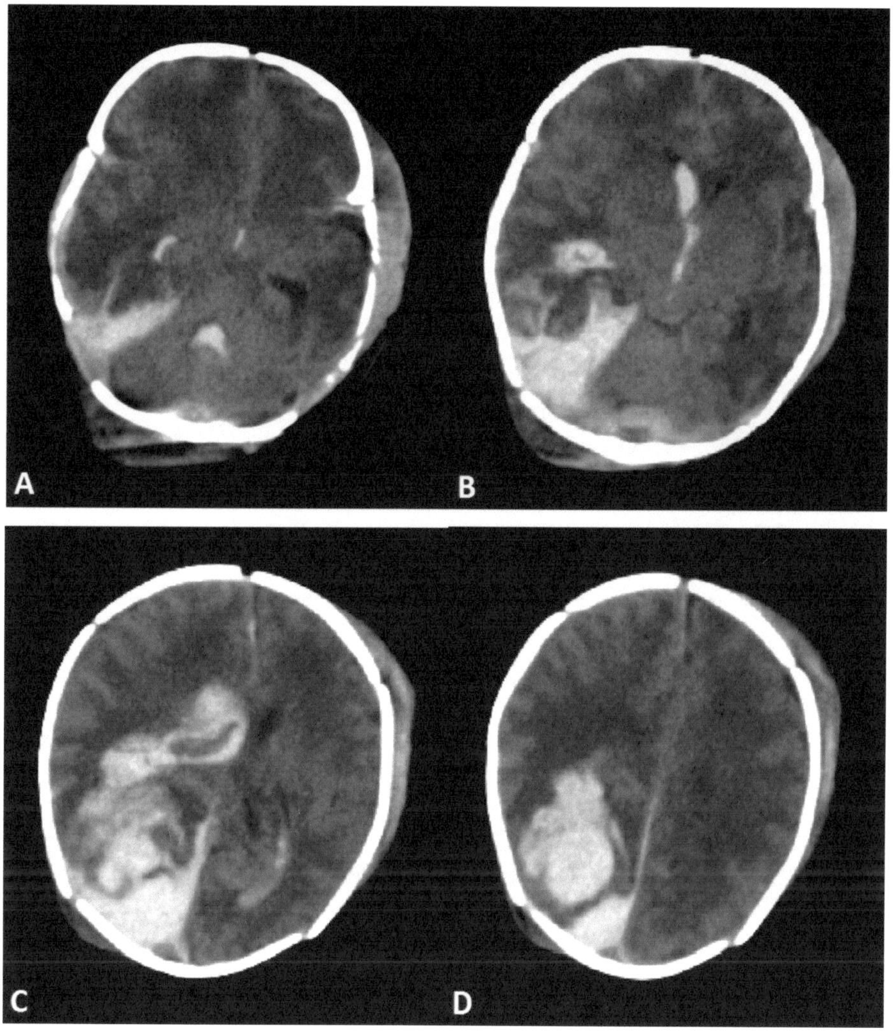

Figure 77.
CT examination of the neonate after severe birth trauma, the first day after birth. Axial sections. Severe intracerebral hemorrhage (parieto-occipital on the right) spread to the ventricular system, hemocephalus without development of acute obstructive hydrocephalus, subdural hematoma above the tentorium on the right, shift of the septum pellucidum by 7 mm to the left, cephalhematoma and swelling of the soft tissues of the skull frontoparietal on the left and parieto-occipital on the right.

velocity in BA was greater than blood flow velocity in the ACA. The value of RI-BA was within normal range. During examination, the characteristic of blood flow in the deep venous system of the brain was not negatively influenced (**Figures 80** and **81**).

Clinical condition of the neonate was stabilized. Seven days after birth, MRI examination of the brain was performed. It did not show any cerebral anomalies or brain tumor. Size of the cerebral ventricles was stabilized. Elimination of midline shift, stability of intracerebral hemorrhage (parieto-occipital right) and subdural hematoma in the tentorium on the right (**Figure 82**) were confirmed. Follow-up treatment in the hospital was without significant changes in the intracranial finding.

15.9 Assessment of intracranial dynamics in the neonate with congenital hydrocephalus and VP shunt revision

The neonate was born in 38th gestation week by cesarean section, with the suspicion to gestational infection of the mother. The postnatal adaptation of the

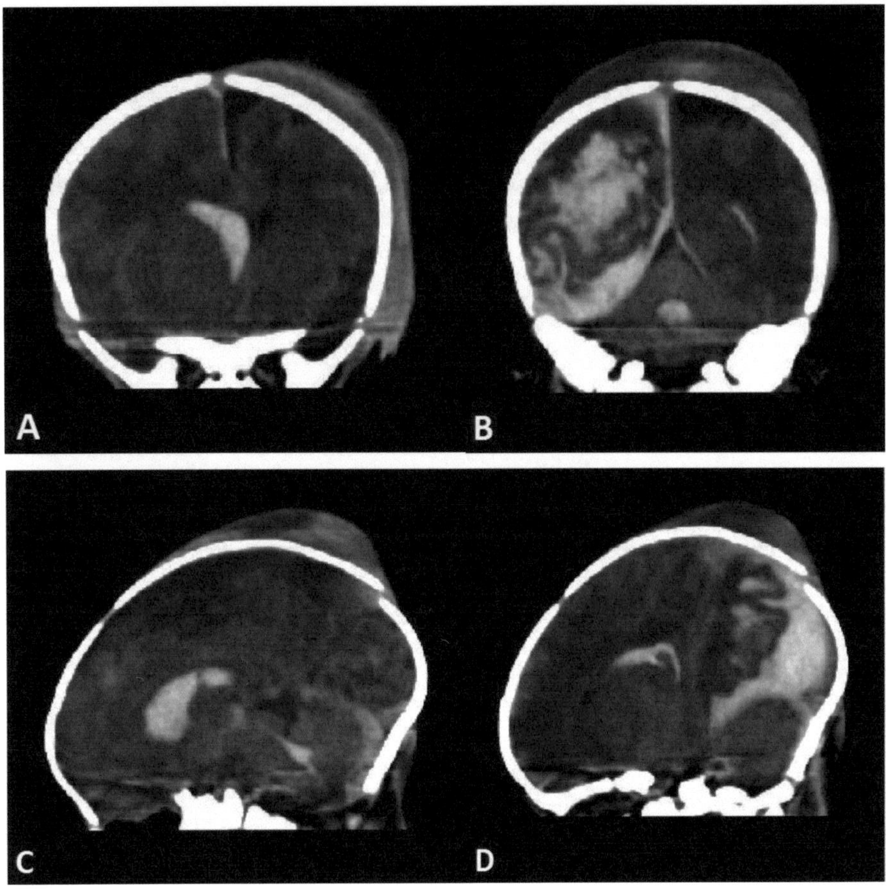

Figure 78.
CT examination of the neonate after severe birth trauma, first day after birth. (A and B) The coronal sections, (C and D) the sagittal sections. Severe intracerebral hemorrhage parieto-occipital on the right spread to the ventricular system, hemocephalus without development of acute obstructive hydrocephalus, subdural hematoma above the tentorium on the right, shift of the septum pellucidum by 7 mm to the left, cephalohematoma and swelling of the soft tissues of the skull, impression of the occipital bone into the intracranial space.

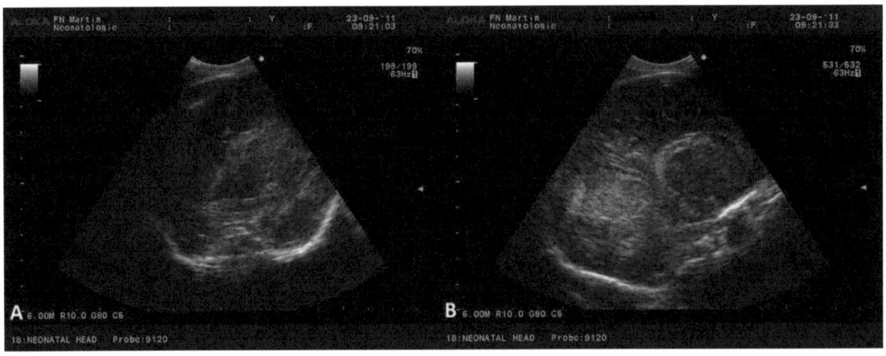

Figure 79.
Sonographic examination of the neonate after severe birth trauma, second day after birth. In comparison with the previous examination, the finding is stationary. (A) coronal plane, (B) sagittal plane.

neonate was appropriate. In the first day after birth, the head circumference of the child was slightly larger, but the intracranial sutures were not enlarged significantly, and the anterior fontanelle was soft when palpated. Significant dilatation of

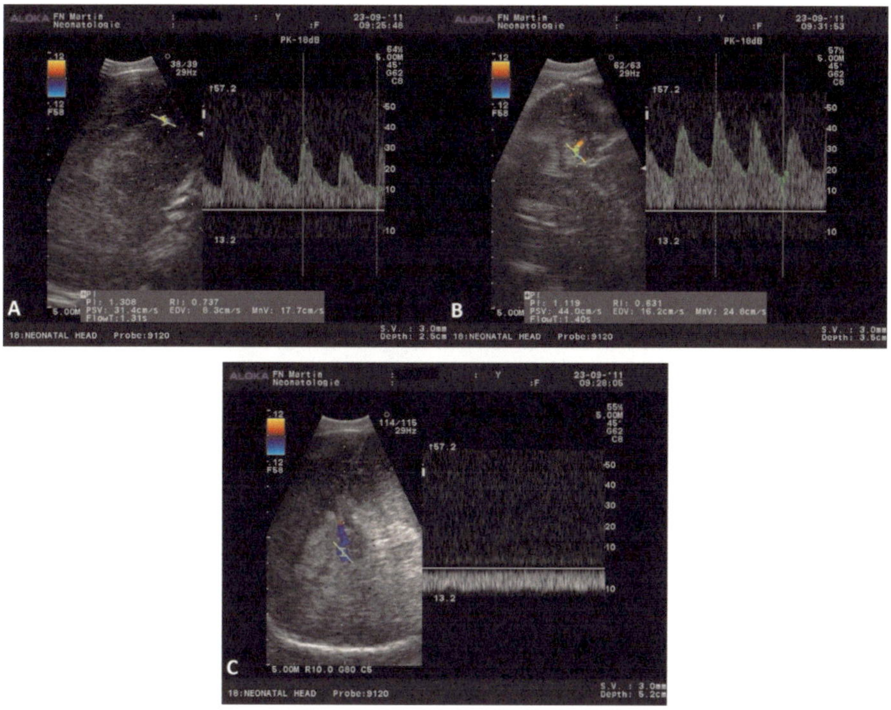

Figure 80.
Examination of cerebral circulation in the neonate after severe birth trauma, second day after birth. (A–sagittal plane, B–coronal plane) Doppler curve of blood flow in ACA, slightly increased RI-ACA, (C) the Doppler curve of blood flow in the internal cerebral vein. Drainage of blood in the deep venous system of the brain was not altered.

the temporal and occipital horns of the lateral cerebral ventricles occurred: WI dx. 13 mm, WI sin. 15.3 mm, VI dx. 20.1 mm, VI sin. 17.9 mm, and width of the third cerebral ventricle 3.8 mm. Doppler parameters of blood flow in ACA were as follows: basal, Vsyst 21.23 cm/s, Ved 6.13 cm/s, RI 0.71, and PI 1.33 (increased RI and PI), and compressive, Vsyst 21.86 cm/s, Ved 0 cm/s, RI 1.0, and PI 2.20 (end-diastolic blockage, positive compressive test).

Thirteen days after birth, MRI of the brain showed three-ventricular hydrocephalus accompanied by stenosis of aqueduct. Significant dilatation of the occipital and temporal horns of the lateral cerebral ventricles was presented. The size of third cerebral ventricle was increased only very slightly. Significant reduction of the cerebral cortex mantle in the occipital region was confirmed (**Figure 83**).

Eighteen days after birth, sonographic examination showed progressive dilatation of the lateral cerebral ventricles, and the width of the third cerebral ventricle had not changed: WI dx. 17.1 mm, WI sin. 17.1 mm, VI dx. 19.9 mm, VI sin. 19.9 mm, and width of the third cerebral ventricle 3.9 mm. Doppler parameters of blood flow in ACA were as follows: basal, Vsyst 30.2 cm/s, Ved 6.4 cm/s, Vmean 15.5 cm/s, RI 0.789, and PI 1.543 (increased RI and PI), and compressive, Vsyst 37.4 cm/s, Ved 0 cm/s, Vmean 18.7 cm/s, RI 0, and PI 2.004 (end-diastolic blockage of blood flow, increased PI, positive compressive test).

Although both MRI and ultrasonography examination of the brain confirmed activity of hydrocephalus (progressive dilatation of the lateral cerebral ventricles, alteration of basal and compressive Doppler parameters, periventricular halo, dominant dilatation in the trigonum, the occipital and temporal horns of the lateral cerebral ventricles), the clinical manifestations were not clear. The cranial sutures

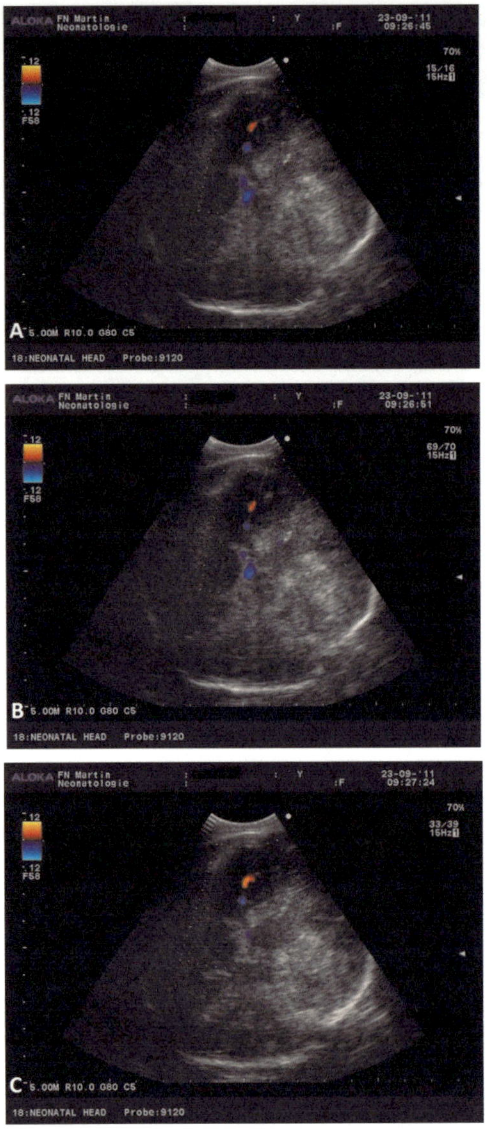

Figure 81.
Examination of cerebral circulation in the neonate after severe birth trauma by transcranial Doppler sonography. The coronal sections (A–C), dislocation of the anterior cerebral artery caused by midline shift to the left.

were only slightly enlarged as well as diameters of the head. The anterior fontanelle was in niveau, boundary finding when palpated. Based on the signs of the activity of hydrocephalus on MRI and sonographic image, the insertion of ventriculoperitoneal shunt was indicated.

Increased value of ICP of 14 cm of CSF column was confirmed by direct measurement during surgery. We can conclude that in this case, excessive accumulation of cerebrospinal fluid due to stenosis of aqueduct and increased ICP led mainly to progressive dilatation of the lateral cerebral ventricles and alteration of Doppler parameters of blood flow in ACA than to clear clinical manifestations of intracranial hypertension. The most likely cause was increased compliance of the brain tissue, which enabled development of significant dilatation of lateral cerebral ventricles. Three days after ventriculoperitoneal shunt insertion, sonographic examination

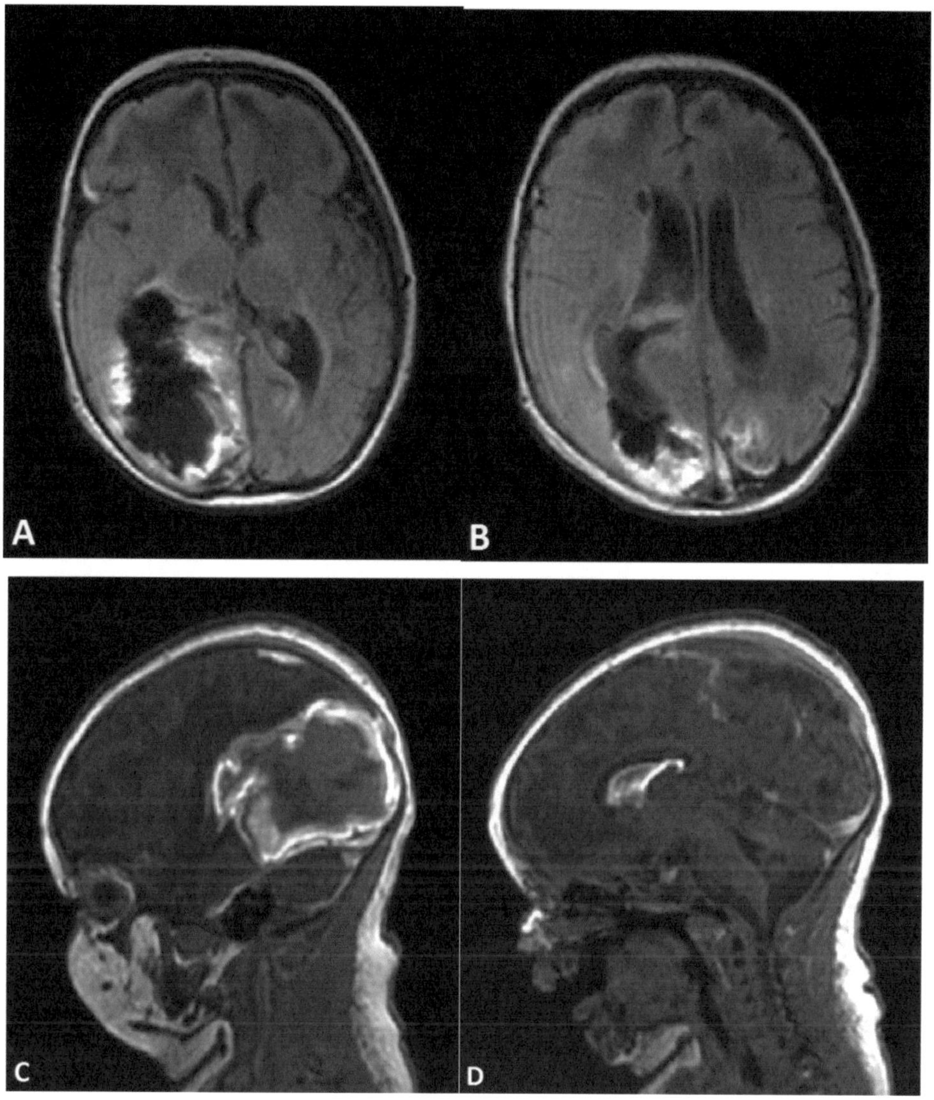

Figure 82.
MRI examination of the brain of the neonate after severe birth trauma, seventh day after birth. In comparison with CT examination of the brain performed in the first day after birth, shift of the midline structures diminished, size of the cerebral ventricles was stable without signs of development of hydrocephalus, and intracerebral hemorrhage (parieto-occipital right) was stable.

showed enlarged lateral cerebral ventricles and the third cerebral ventricle: WI dx. 11.5 mm, WI sin. 11.4 mm, VI dx. 20.3 mm, VI sin. 19.1 mm, and width of the third cerebral ventricle 2 mm. Also, changes in Doppler parameters of blood flow in ACA were measured: basal, Vsyst 42.63 cm/s, Ved 16.52 cm/s, RI 0.61, and PI 0.90 (decreased RI due to increased Ved), and compressive, Vsyst 49.74 cm/s, Ved 15.93 cm/s, RI 0.68, and PI 1.1 (negative compressive test).

Retroauricular subcutaneous CSF accumulation occurred after 3 weeks. It enlarged when baby was crying and diminished at the rest. As retroauricular subcutaneous CSF accumulation has been growing (**Figure 84**), whole-body X-ray focused on drainage system function, X-ray of the skull (**Figure 85**), and CT examination of the brain were performed. The examinations showed dislocation of the ventricular catheter from intracranial space beyond the calva (**Figure 86**).

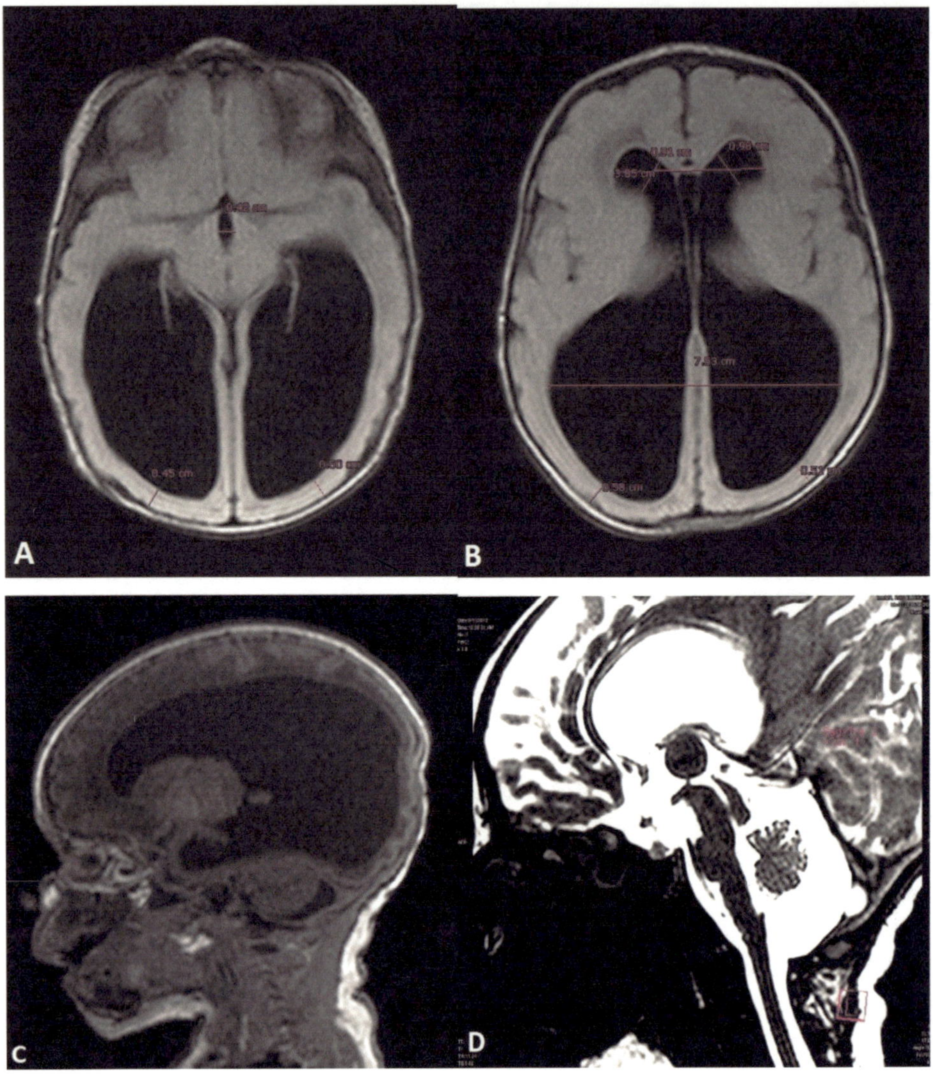

Figure 83.
MRI examination of the brain of the neonate with congenital three-ventricular hydrocephalus. (A and B) The axial sections, significant dilatation of cerebral ventricles accompanied only mild dilatation of the third cerebral ventricle, (C) the sagittal section, significant dilatation in the trigonum and occipital horn of the lateral cerebral ventricle, (D) the high-resolution sequence for assessment of the aqueduct blockage, confirmation of aqueduct stenosis.

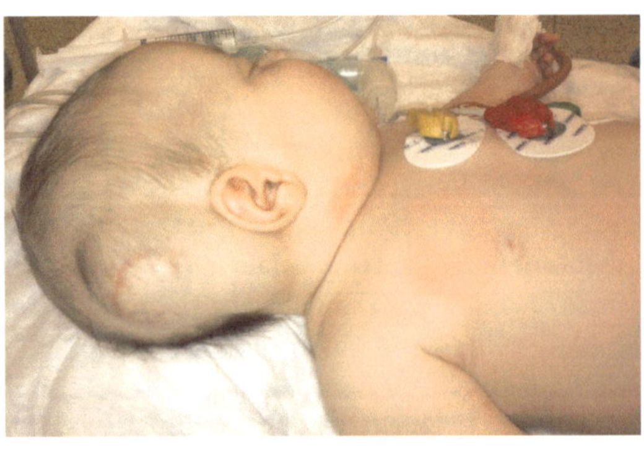

Figure 84.
Dysfunction of ventriculoperitoneal shunt in the child with hydrocephalus. Manifestation of subcutaneous cerebrospinal fluid accumulation.

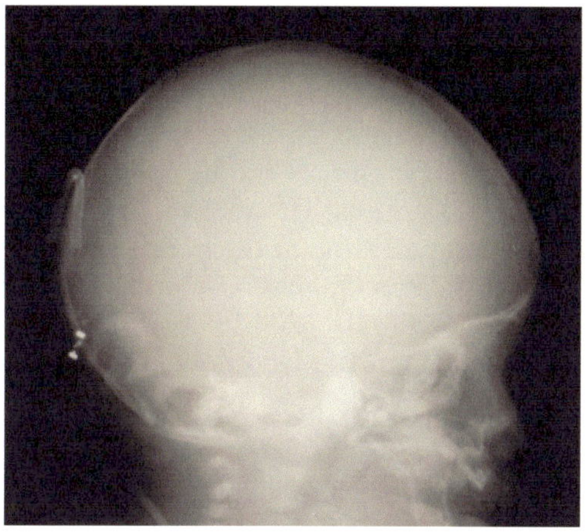

Figure 85.
X-ray image of the skull of the child with hydrocephalus, dysfunction of ventriculoperitoneal shunt. Presence of dislocation of ventricular catheter from the intracranial space beyond the calva.

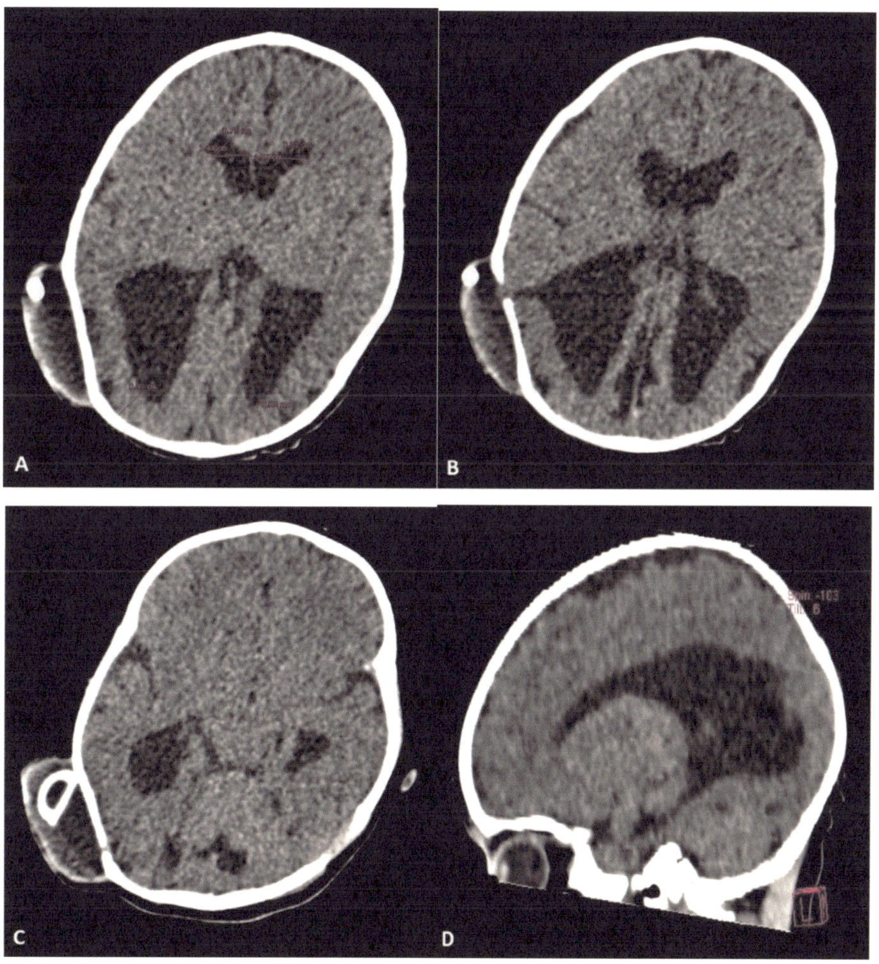

Figure 86.
CT examination of the brain of the child with hydrocephalus, dysfunction of ventriculoperitoneal shunt. (A, B, and C) The axial sections, presence of subcutaneous CSF accumulation, the shunt "flowing" freely in the subcutaneous collection, the small trepanation whole in the calva, and the channel in the brain tissue enable CSF drainage from the cerebral ventricle into the subcutaneous space, decrease of the size of the cerebral ventricles, and thickening of the cerebral mantle (compared to MRI image before shunt insertion), (D) sagittal section, decreased dilatation of the lateral cerebral ventricle.

Basal Doppler parameters of blood flow in ACA were within the standard range: Vsyst 64 cm/s, Ved 21.2 cm/s, and RI 0.67. Compressive test was not performed because of the small size of the anterior fontanelle. CT examination of the brain showed decrease of the lateral cerebral ventricles and thickening of the cerebral cortex mantle. There were not any clinical manifestations of intracranial hypertension nor diastasis of the cranial sutures. The anterior fontanelle was small and soft when palpated. Regarding compensation of the intracranial space, cerebrospinal fluid drainage through a small trepanation whole in the calva to the subcutaneous space was effective. This resulted in decreased size of the cerebral ventricles and normal range of Doppler parameters of blood flow in ACA. Blockage of the valve

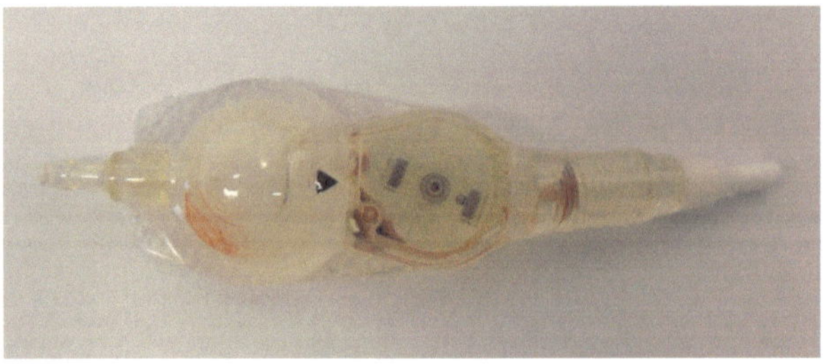

Figure 87.
The blocked programmable CODMAN®CERTAS™valve. The valve obstruction caused by blood sediment.

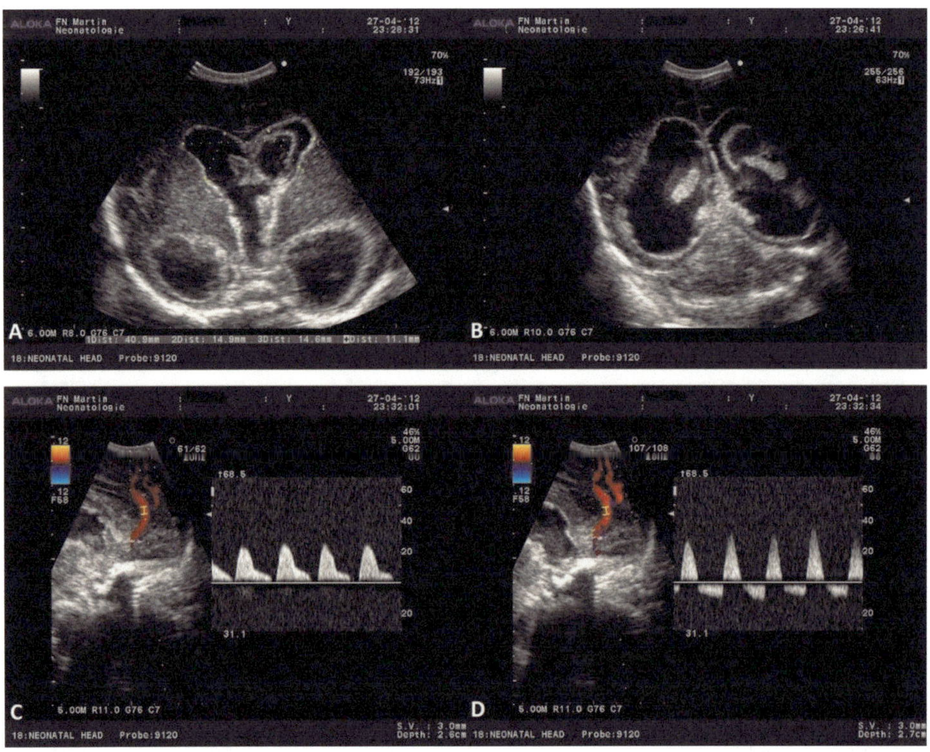

Figure 88.
Sonographic examination of the brain of the neonate with congenital postinfectious hydrocephalus, performed 1 hour after birth. (A and B) Significant dilatation of the lateral cerebral ventricles and the third cerebral ventricle, hyperechogenicity of the wall of the cerebral ventricles and the choroid plexus, hemorrhage in the lateral cerebral ventricles, reduction of the cerebral mantle in the occipital region of the brain, (C) alteration of basal and compressive Doppler parameters of blood flow in ACA, (D) positive compressive test on the anterior fontanelle with reverse blood flow during diastole.

was confirmed during revision surgery (**Figure 87**). Obstruction of the valve of drainage system disabled drainage of cerebrospinal fluid through the shunt. It resulted in the rise of intracranial pressure, which was followed by pushing the ventricular catheter out of the intracranial space beyond the calva. When cerebrospinal fluid drainage had been performed through the small trepanation whole in the calva, intracranial pressure dropped down.

This case study shows that dynamics of dilatation of cerebral ventricles and Doppler parameters of blood flow in ACA represent the state of compensation of the intracranial space in respect to pressure-volume changes but not the drainage system dysfunction itself. After surgery, the child's condition was stable without relapse of subcutaneous CSF accumulation, and wound was healing well. Basal Doppler parameters of blood flow in ACA were within the normal range: Vsyst 63.8 cm/s, Ved 21.0 cm/s, and RI 0.671.

15.10 Assessment of intracranial dynamics of congenital hydrocephalus in prenatal and postnatal period

Dilatation of cerebral ventricles was detected by prenatal sonographic examination in the fetus in 33rd gestation week. Up to then, gestation was without complications and without any signs of maternal infection. Prenatal sonographic examination performed 1 week later, in 34th gestation week, confirmed significant progression of dilatation of the lateral cerebral ventricles and reduction of the

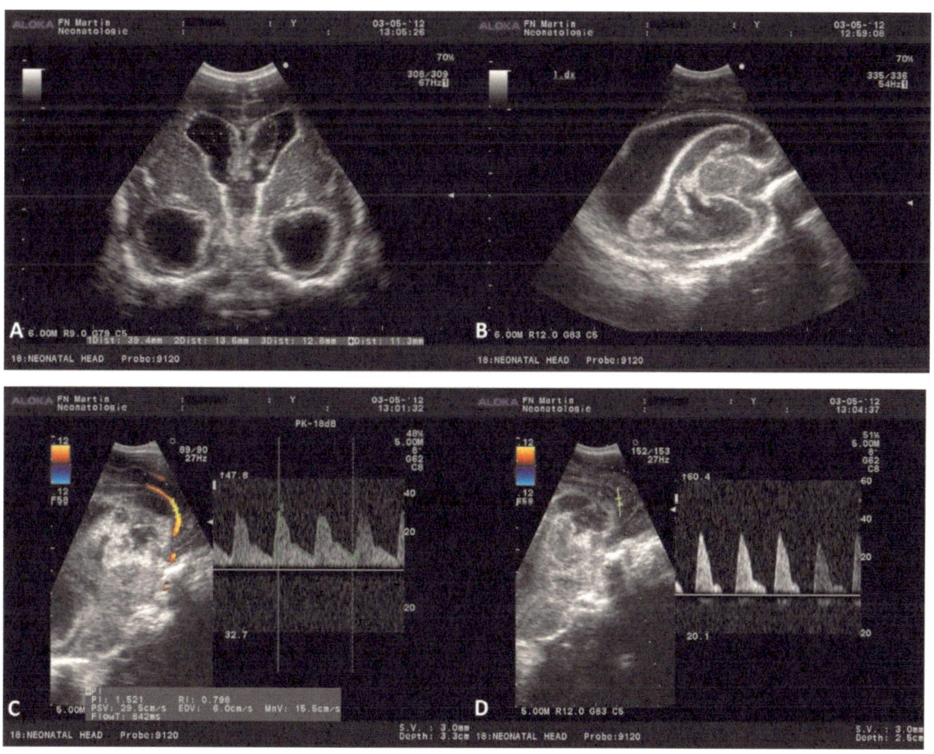

Figure 89.
Stable finding of the brain taken by sonography 2 days after ventricular puncture and cerebrospinal fluid derivation in the neonate with congenital postinfectious hydrocephalus. (A) The coronal section, morphometry of the cerebral ventricles, (B) the sagittal section, dilatation of the right lateral cerebral ventricle with hemorrhage, (C) the normal range of Doppler parameters of blood flow in ACA, (D) negative compressive test on the anterior fontanelle.

cerebral mantle, especially in the occipital region of the brain. Because progression was rapid, prenatal interdisciplinary consultation between the gynecologist-obstetrician, neonatologist, and neurosurgeon and then appointment with parents were arranged. Preterm labor was indicated so that early drainage procedure could be performed. Cesarean section was performed without any complications. Neurosurgeon examined the child 1 hour after birth. The first postnatal sonographic examination of the brain was performed. Increased head circumference, diastasis of cranial sutures, and tense anterior fontanelle were presented in the clinical picture. Sonographic examination of the brain showed significant dilatation of the lateral cerebral ventricles and the third cerebral ventricle, hyperechogenicity of the choroidal plexus, and hemorrhage in the lateral cerebral ventricles. High echogenicity of the wall of the cerebral ventricles indicated ventriculitis. Also, alteration of basal and compressive Doppler parameters of blood flow in ACA was confirmed (**Figure 88**). Ventricular puncture was performed because clinical and sonographic signs indicated activity of hydrocephalus. The value of ICP was 11.5 of CSF column (macroscopically brown-green); after derivation of 20 ml of cerebrospinal fluid, ICP dropped to 3 cm of CSF column. Also, the anterior fontanelle changed to soft when palpated. Biochemical examination of cerebrospinal fluid confirmed increased concentration of proteins and number of erythrocytes. The values of C-reactive protein and procalcitonin in serum of the neonate were in normal range. In the mother's blood, positive IgG antibodies against toxoplasmosis were found,

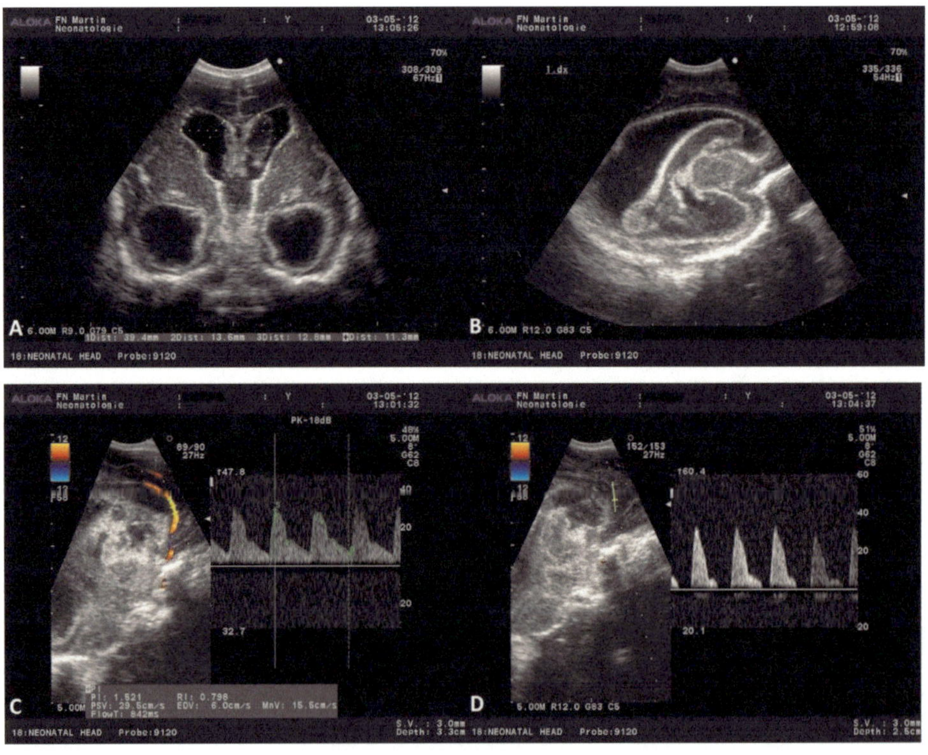

Figure 90.
Sonographic examination of the brain of the neonate with congenital postinfectious hydrocephalus, fifth day after birth. (A) The coronal section, stable size of the cerebral ventricles, (B) the sagittal section, the stable dilatation of the right lateral cerebral ventricle with hemorrhage, (C) alteration of basal Doppler parameters of blood flow in ACA, increased RI, (D) positive compressive test on the anterior fontanelle with end-diastolic blockage of blood flow in ACA.

which indicated overcoming of toxoplasmosis during gestation. From an etiological perspective, the condition was diagnosed as congenital postinfectious hydrocephalus with hemorrhage in the lateral cerebral ventricles due to overcoming intrauterine toxoplasmic neuroinfection.

Dynamics of hydrocephalus was assessed daily by clinical examination and transcranial sonography of the brain as well as by assessing Doppler parameters of blood flow in ACA (**Figure 89**). One-time early postnatal puncture of the cerebral ventricle with cerebrospinal fluid derivation maintained compensation of hydrocephalus during 4 days and so enabled biochemical and microbiological assessment of cerebrospinal fluid as well as stabilizing of extracranial factors.

Five days after birth, head circumference had increased, and finding on the anterior fontanelle had changed (bulged, tense when palpated); the cranial sutures had been enlarged. The sonographic image did not show progression of dilatation of the cerebral ventricles. Despite the stable dilatation of the cerebral ventricles, alteration of Doppler parameters of blood flow in ACA was found (**Figure 90**). Subcutaneous reservoir insertion and regular cerebrospinal fluid derivation were indicated. The regime of daily liquor derivation of 24 ml from subcutaneous reservoir ensured compensation of hydrocephalus and positive change of Doppler parameters of blood flow in ACA (**Figure 91**). Ventriculoperitoneal shunt insertion was performed on the 27th day after birth.

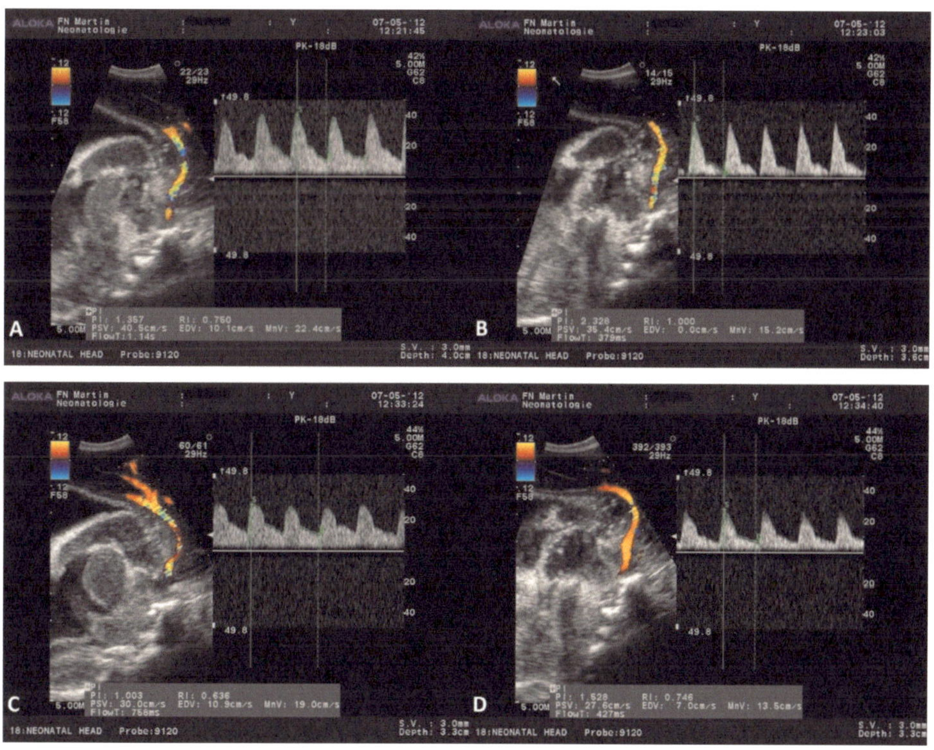

Figure 91.
Examination of blood flow in ACA by transcranial Doppler ultrasonography before and after CSF derivation from subcutaneous reservoir in the neonate with congenital postinfectious hydrocephalus. (A) Alteration of basal Doppler parameters (increased RI and PI) before CSF derivation, (B) the positive compressive test on the anterior fontanelle with end-diastolic blockage of blood flow before CSF derivation, (C) improvement of basal Doppler parameters within the normal range after CSF derivation (decreased RI and PI), (D) the negative compressive test on the anterior fontanelle with end-diastolic blockage of blood flow after CSF derivation.

16. Report of assessment of intracranial dynamics in neonate and infant with hydrocephalus

Patient's name:
Date of birth:
DG.:
Etiology of hydrocephalus:
Date of examination:
Time relation to drainage procedure:
General condition of a patient on examination: ⤡sleeping ⤡calm ⤡crying
Analgesics sedation: No Yes: ____________________________

I. Clinical manifestations

• Diastasis of cranial sutures	Yes	No	
• Diastasis of sagittal suture	Yes	No	
• Diastasis of lambdoid suture	Yes	No	
• Palpated finding on the anterior fontanelle			
o Soft	Yes	No	
o Boundary tense	Yes	No	
o Tense, bulged	Yes	No	
• Head circumference increased the same progression regression stable			
• Sunset eyes syndrome	Yes	No	
• Vomiting	Yes	No	
• Breathing pattern disorders, apneic pauses	Yes	No	
• Bradycardia	Yes	No	
• Apathy, somnolence	Yes	No	
• Hypersensitivity	Yes	No	
• Drainage system:	Yes	No	
o Type of drainage procedure			
o Palpable functional valve	Yes	No	Not clear
o Other			
• Drainage functioning Functional Dysfunctional			
• Cause of drainage dysfunction			
• Subcutaneous CSF accumulation, CSF fistula, CSF leak	Yes	No	
• Associated disorders, pathological conditions			

Ophthalmologic examination:

• Examination of ocular background	Yes	No
• Presence of edema in the optic disc	Yes	No

- Presence of atrophy in the optic disc Yes No
- Other ophthalmologic findings

II. **Extracranial factors** Stable Nonstable

- Hematocrit Hemoglobin Heart rate Blood pressure
- Acidobasis S_aO2 p_aO2 p_aCO2 pH
- Pulse oximeter S_pO2
- Body temperature
- Mechanical ventilation Yes No Type of ventilation

III. **USG examination of the brain**

- Dilatation of cerebral ventricles Yes No
- Dynamics of dilatation of cerebral ventricles Stable Progression Regression
- Asymmetric dilatation of the lateral cerebral ventricles Yes No
- Shift of midlines structures Yes No
- Type of hydrocephalus
- Width (WI) of the frontal horn of the lateral cerebral ventricle Left: Right:
- Ventricular index (VI) of the frontal horn of the lateral ventricle Left: Right:
- Width (WI) of the third cerebral ventricle
- Width (WI) of the fourth cerebral ventricle
- Periventricular leukomalacia, cysts Yes No
- Other pathological findings:

IV. **TCCD examination of the brain: the segment of ACA before the genu corporis callosi in the sagittal section**

Basal parameters

- Vsyst Ved Vmean
- RI (Pourcelot) PI (Gösling)

Compressive parameters

- Vsyst Ved Vmean
- RI (Pourcelot) PI (Gösling)

V. **CT and MRI examination of the brain**

- Type of hydrocephalus
- Periventricular edema Yes No

- Width (WI) of the frontal horn of the lateral cerebral ventricle Left: Right:
- Ventricular index (VI) of the frontal horn of the lateral ventricle Left: Right:
- Width (WI) of the third cerebral ventricle
- Width (WI) of the fourth cerebral ventricle
- Evans' index
- Frontal-occipital horn ratio (FOR)
- Other pathological findings:

VI. **Assessment of the condition, notes, and conclusion**

17. Conclusions

Healthcare about the child with hydrocephalus gradually develops using the latest knowledge and its application in clinical practice. Milestone in treatment of pediatric hydrocephalus in the middle of last century was determined by the use of drainage systems with a valve mechanism which enabled regulated internal cerebrospinal drainage. Since then, new and modern valves have been developed to ensure physiological alternative drainage of cerebrospinal fluid as much as possible. Despite that, shunt insertion is related to infectious and noninfectious conditions, which have a negative effect on psychomotor development of the child. The second milestone has been more frequent implementation of endoscopic methods in treatment of children with hydrocephalus since the end of last century.

Assessment of a child with hydrocephalus should be based on understanding pathophysiology and biomechanics of hydrocephalus. Therefore, the research is focused on assessment of intracranial dynamics and analysis of pressure-volume relationships, which are combined with assessment of intracranial pressure and compliance. Transcranial Doppler ultrasonography has been used as a noninvasive technique for indirect measurement of intracranial pressure and effect of drainage surgery because it enables to assess values of blood flow velocity in the cerebral arteries and cerebrovascular resistance. In general, increased intracranial pressure leads to increased cerebrovascular resistance of the cerebral arteries. This results in increased resistance index and pulsatility index of the Doppler curve of blood flow in the cerebral arteries. Initial discrepancy in methodology of the use of transcranial Doppler ultrasonography and interpretation of data resulted in various conclusions. Since then, various research studies have brought precisely defined methodology and analysis of Doppler parameters of cerebral circulation. Complex relationship between size of cerebral ventricles, intracranial pressure, intracranial compliance, and Doppler parameters of cerebral circulation, accompanied by impact of multiple intra- and extracranial factors on cerebral circulation, is responsible for the condition that not in each case the values of measured Doppler parameters reflect automatically the increased value of intracranial pressure. This fact is one of the causes why assessment of cerebral circulation by transcranial Doppler ultrasonography in children with hydrocephalus remains to be open for discussion.

Based on our (the author of this monography) 17-year-long clinical experience and scientific research on pediatric hydrocephalus, we can summarize the results of research and a role of transcranial Doppler ultrasonography in assessment of intracranial dynamics of pediatric hydrocephalus as follows:

1. Assessment of Doppler parameters of cerebral circulation before drainage procedure in children with hydrocephalus revealed alteration of basal and compressive parameters of the Doppler curve of blood flow in ACA. Increased RI-ACA was caused by decreased Ved [389, 436]. After drainage procedure, RI-ACA values dropped down to the normal range because of increased values of Ved. Change of Doppler parameters before and after drainage procedure confirmed positive effect of the drainage procedure to cerebral circulation in children with hydrocephalus [319, 320, 387].

2. Realization of compressive test on the anterior fontanelle during sonographic examination increases validity of assessment of cerebral circulation by transcranial Doppler ultrasonography and enables indirect assessment of decrease of intracranial compliance. Increase of basal Doppler parameters reflects increase of intracranial pressure [289].

3. While interpreting Doppler parameters of cerebral circulation measured in a child with hydrocephalus, it is important to assess impact of both intra- and extracranial factors on cerebral circulation. Then it is possible to say to which extent Doppler parameters show the real value of intracranial pressure and intracranial compliance. The fact is that extracranial factors affect cerebral circulation. Our research was focused on detailed analysis of impact of the intracranial morphologic factors on Doppler parameters of blood flow in ACA. The results showed that asymmetric dilatation of the lateral cerebral ventricles and posthemorrhagic periventricular lesions influenced the RI-ACA values both in intracranial hypertension and intracranial normotension [319].

4. While assessing relation between dynamics of dilatation of the cerebral ventricles and value of RI-ACA, we found out that the values of RI-ACA were increased in those cases in which stable dilatation of the cerebral ventricles was accompanied by increased intracranial pressure and drainage procedure was necessary. On the contrary, the values of RI-ACA were within the normal range in children in which intracranial pressure wasn't increased. The results show that the values of RI-ACA in active hydrocephalus aren't increased due to dilatation of cerebral ventricles but increased intracranial pressure [319, 400].

5. Assessment of Doppler parameters of blood flow in ACA in children with hydrocephalus with functional drainage system or ETV revealed normal range of RI-ACA values. On the other hand, the values of RI-ACA increased in the shunt-dependent children with dysfunctional drainage system and ETV, even though the cerebral ventricles enlarged slightly or maintained the same size. After successful revision surgery, the value of RI-ACA dropped down to normal range [319, 320, 387].

6. Assessment of cerebral circulation by transcranial Doppler ultrasonography in children with hydrocephalus allows an accessible, indirect, noninvasive, bedside, and repetitive measurement of intracranial pressure and intracranial compliance. Regarding complexity of intracranial dynamics, the relationship between intracranial pressure and Doppler parameters of the cerebral arteries, individual assessment of measured Doppler parameters, as well as assessment of effect of extra- and intracranial factors to cerebral circulation should be performed in each case of pediatric hydrocephalus. If the results are not clear, examination should be repeated, and intraindividual tendency

should be observed in the child. It is important to design and follow detailed methodology of sonographic examination and include it into the report of assessment of intracranial dynamics in the child with hydrocephalus [186, 266, 289].

7. Clinical applications of transcranial Doppler ultrasonography in children with hydrocephalus are as follows [289]:

   - Indication and timing of drainage procedure
   - Observation of effectivity of drainage procedure—internal drainage systems (shunts), ventriculostomy of the third cerebral ventricle, external ventricular drainage, cerebrospinal fluid derivation from subcutaneous Rickham reservoir (determination of frequency and amount of aspired cerebrospinal fluid)
   - Observation of function and detection of malfunction of external and internal drainage systems and ventriculostomy of the third cerebral ventricle
   - Assessment of dependence of the child on drainage system (shunt dependence)—important for indication of external ventricular drainage conversion, Rickham reservoir conversion on internal drainage system (shunt), and ETV, need for a revision of dysfunctional drainage system.

To sum up, it can be said that including assessment of cerebral circulation by transcranial Doppler ultrasonography into management of children with hydrocephalus provides additional information to clinical manifestation and morphological results of imaging techniques. This helps better understand intracranial dynamics and activity of hydrocephalus in regard to indication and timing of drainage procedure.

Abbreviations

ACA	anterior cerebral artery
aEEG	amplitude electroencephalography
AT	acceleration time
ATP	adenosine triphosphate, adenosine triphosphate acid
BA	basilar artery
C	compliance
cAMP	cyclic adenosine triphosphate
CBF	cerebral blood flow
CDE	color Doppler energy
CFD	color flow Doppler
cGMP	cyclic guanosine monophosphate
cm/s	centimeter per second
CNS	central nervous system
CO_2	carbon dioxide
COX-1	cyclooxygenase 1
COX-2	cyclooxygenase 2
CPA	color power angio
CPP	cerebral perfusion pressure

CSF	cerebrospinal fluid
CT	computed tomography
CVR	cerebrovascular resistance
CW	continuous wave
DWM	Dandy-Walker malformation
DWS	Dandy-Walker syndrome
eNOS	endothelial synthetase of nitric oxide
EPO	erythropoietin
ET	endothelin
ETV	endoscopic third ventriculostomy
EVD	external ventricular drainage
FHR	frontal horn ratio
FOR	frontal/occipital horn ratio
g	gram
g/cm^2	gram per square centimeter
GABA	gamma-aminobutyric acid
GLAST	glutamate/aspartate transport system
H^+	hydrogen cations
H_2O	water
Hz	hertz, unit of frequency
ICA	internal carotid artery
ICP	intracranial pressure
ICV	internal cerebral vein
ICH	intracranial hypertension
iNOS	induced synthetase of nitric oxide
IOR	index of regulation
IRDS	idiopathic respiratory distress syndrome
IV	interventricular distance
IVH	intraventricular hemorrhage
K^+	potassium cations
kg	kilogram
lCBF	local cerebral blood flow
m/s	meter per second
m^3	cubic meter
MAP	mean arterial pressure
MCA	middle cerebral artery
MHz	megahertz
min	minute
ml	milliliter
MR spectroscopy	magnetic resonance spectroscopy
MRI	magnetic resonance imaging
mW/cm^2	milliwatt per square centimeter
Na	natrium
NGF	nerve growth factor
nNOS	neural synthetase of nitric oxide
NO	nitric oxide
NOS	synthetase of nitric oxide
O_2	oxygen
p_aCO_2	partial arterial blood pressure of carbon dioxide
p_aO_2	partial arterial blood pressure of oxygen
PCA	posterior cerebral artery
PDA	ductus arteriosus Botalli apertus
PHH	posthemorrhagic hydrocephalus

PI	index of pulsatility, Gösling's index
PRF	pulsed repetitive frequency
PW	pulsed wave
Re	Reynold's number
RI	index of resistance, Pourcelot's index
S/D index	systolic/diastolic index
SVP	synaptic vesicle protein
TC	transcerebral distance
TCCD	transcranial color-coded Doppler sonography
tRNA	transcription ribonucleic acid
USG	ultrasonography
VA	vertebral artery
Ved	end-diastolic blood flow velocity
VEGF	vascular endothelial growth factor
VIdx.	ventricular index of right lateral cerebral ventricle
VIsin.	ventricular index of left lateral cerebral ventricle
Vmean	mean blood flow velocity
VP shunt	ventriculoperitoneal shunt
Vsyst	peak systolic blood flow velocity
W/cm^2	watt per square centimeter
Wdx.	width of the right lateral cerebral ventricle
Wsin.	width of the left lateral cerebral ventricle

Author details

Branislav Kolarovszki
Clinic of Neurosurgery, Jessenius Faculty of Medicine in Martin, Comenius University in Bratislava, University Hospital Martin, Slovakia

*Address all correspondence to: branislav.kolarovszki@uniba.sk

References

[1] Čihák R. Liquor cerebrospinalis—mozkomíšní mok. In: Čihák R Anatomie 3. Praha: Grada Publishing; 1997. pp. 293-294

[2] Sweadner KJ, Gilkeson RC. Two isoenzymes of the Na,K-ATP-ase have distinct antigenic determinants. The Journal of Biological Chemistry. 1985; **260**:9016-9022

[3] Johanson CE. Potential for pharmacologic manipulation of the blood-cerebrospinal fluid barrier. In: Neuwelt EA, editor. Implications of the Blood-Brain Barrier and Its Manipulation. Vol. 1. New York: Plenum Press; 1989. p. 403

[4] McComb JG. Recent research into the nature of cerebrospinal fluid formation and absorption. Journal of Neurosurgery. 1983;**59**:369-383

[5] Sainte-Rose C. Hydrocephalus in childhood. In: Youmans JR, editor. Neurosurgical Surgery. Vol. 2. Philadelphia: W.B. Saunders Company; 1996. pp. 890-926

[6] Greenberg MS. Handbook of Neurosurgery. 4th ed. Vol. II. Lakeland, Florida: Greenberg Graphics, Inc.; 1997. pp. 571-600

[7] McCarthy KD, Reed DJ. The effect of acetazolamide and furosemide on cerebrospinal fluid production and choroid plexus carnonic anhydrase activity. The Journal of Pharmacology and Experimental Therapeutics. 1974; **189**:194-201

[8] Sahar A, Tsipstein E. Effects of mannitol and furosemide on the rate of formation of cerebrospinal fluid. Experimental Neurology. 1978;**60**: 584-591

[9] Sato O, Bering EA. Extraventricular formation of cerebrospinal fluid. Brain and Nerve. 1967;**19**:883-885

[10] Available from: http://www.totalhealth.co.uk/clinical-experts/mr-christopher-chandler/hydrocephalus

[11] Hadač J. Ultrazvukové vyšetření mozku přes velkou fontanelu. Praha: Triton; 2000. p. 197

[12] Kida S, Yamashima T, Kubota T, Ito H, Yamamoto S. A light and electron microscopy and immunohistochemical study of human arachnoid villi. Journal of Neurosurgery. 1988;**69**:429-435

[13] Odio C, Mohs E, Sklar FH, Nelson JD, McCracken GH Jr. Adverse reactions to vancomycin used as prophylactis for CSF shunt procedures. American Journal of Diseases of Children. 1984;**138**:17-19

[14] Tripathi RC. Ultrastructure of the arachnoid mater in relation to outflow of cerebrospinal fluid: A new concept. Lancet. 1973;**2**:8-11

[15] Yamashima T. Ultrastructural study of the final cerebrospinal fluid pathway in human arachnoid villi. Brain Research. 1986;**384**:68-76

[16] Griffith HB, Jamjoom AB. The treatment of childhood hydrocephalus by choroid plexus coagulation and artifitial cerebrospinal fluid perfusion. British Journal of Neurosurgery. 1990;**4**: 95-100

[17] Pierre-Kahn A, Gabersek V, Hirsch JF. Intracranial pressure and rapid eye movement sleep in hydrocephalus. Child's Brain. 1976;**2**: 156-166

[18] Sainte-Rose C, Lacombe J, Pierre-Kahn A, Renier D, Hirsch JF. Intracranial venous sinus hypertension: Cause or consequence of hydrocephalus in infants? Journal of Neurosurgery. 1984;**60**:727-736

[19] Monro A. Observation on the structure and the function of the nervous system. Creek Johnson, Edinburgh. Dotlač: Monro A (2010) Observations on the Structure and Functions of the Nervous System Illustrated with Tables by Alexander Monro. BiblioBazaar; 1783. p. 240

[20] Kellie G. An account of the appearance observed in the dissection of two of three individuals presumed to have perished in the storm of the 3D and whose bodies were discovered in the vinicity of Leith on the morning of the 4th November 1821, with some reflections on the pathology of the brain. Transactions. Medico-Chirurgical Society of Edinburgh. 1824;**84**:1

[21] Available from: http://findmeacure.com/2011/07/25/hydrocephalus-2/hydrocephalus-2/

[22] Kolarovszki B, Šutovský J, Ďurdík P, De Riggo J. Etiopatogenéza a biomechanika detského hydrocefalu. Pediatria. 2006;**1**:84-87

[23] Smrčka M. Poranění mozku. Praha: Grada Publishing; 2001. p. 278

[24] Bloomfield I, Bilston L. Effect of biochemical composition on cerebrospinal fluid viscosity. In: Advaces in Bioengineering, Proceedings of the ASME International Mechnical Engineering Congress; Anaheim, USA. 1998. pp. 357-358

[25] Bloomfield I, Bilston L, Johnston I. Effects of proteins, blood cells and glucose on the viscosity of cerebrospinal fluid. Pediatric Neurosurgery. 1998;**28**:246-251

[26] Symon L. A comparative study od midle cerebral pressure in dogs and macaques. The Journal of Physiology. 1967;**191**:448

[27] Tsuji M, Saul JP, du Plessis A, Eichenwald E, Sobh J, Crocker R, et al. Cerebral intravascular oxygenation correlates with mean arterial pressure in critically ill premature infants. Pediatrics. 2000;**106**:625-632

[28] Volpe JJ. Neurology of the Newborn. 4th ed. Vol. 2001. Philadelphia: WB Saunders; 2001. p. 428

[29] Volpe JJ, Herscovitch P, Perlman JM, Kreusser KL, Raichle ME. Positron emission tomography in the asphyxiated term newborn: Parasagital impairment of cerebral blood flow. Annals of Neurology. 1985;**17**:287-296

[30] Krägeloh-Mann I, Toft P, Lunding J, Andersen J, Pryds O, Lou HC. Brain lesions in preterm: Origin, consequences and compensation. Acta Paediatrica. 1999;**88**:897-908

[31] Kehrer M, Krägeloh-Mann I, Goelz R, Schöning M. The development of cerebral perfusion in healthy preterm and term neonates. Neuropediatrics. 2003;**34**:281-286

[32] Kinnala A, Suhonen Polvi H, Äärimaa T, Kero P, Korvenranta H, Ruotsalainen U, et al. Cerebral metabolic rate for glocose during the first six months of live: An FDG positron emission tomography study. Archives of Disease in Childhood. Fetal and Neonatal Edition. 1996;**74**:F153-F157

[33] Yoxall CW, Weindling AM. Measurement of cerebral oxygen consumption in the human neonate using near infrared spectroscopy: Cerebral oxygen consumption increases with advancing gestational age. Pediatric Research. 1998;**44**:283-290

[34] Hüppi PS, Warfield S, Kikinis R, Barnes PD, Zientara GP, Jolesz FA, et al. Quantitative magnetic resonance imaging of brain development in premature and mature newborns. Annals of Neurology. 1998;**43**:224-235

[35] Børch K, Greisen G. Blood flow distribution in the normal human preterm brain. Pediatric Research. 1998; **43**:28-33

[36] Scheel P, Ruge C, Petruch UR, Schöning M. Color duplex measurement of cerebral blood flow volume in healthy adults. Stroke. 2000;**31**:147-150

[37] Schöning M, Hartig B. Age dependence of total cerebral blood flow volume from childhood to adulthood. Journal of Cerebral Blood Flow and Metabolism. 1996;**16**:827-833

[38] Döfler P, Puls I, Schliesser M, Mäurer M, Becker G. Measurement of cerebral blood flow volume by extracranial sonography. Journal of Cerebral Blood Flow and Metabolism. 2000;**20**:269-271

[39] Schöning M, Staab M, Walter J. Transcranial color duplex sonography in childhood and adolescence, age dependence of flow velocities and waveform parameters. Stroke. 1993;**14**: 1305-1309

[40] Schöning M, Walter J, Scheel P. Estimation of cerebral blood flow through color duplex sonography of the carotid and vertebral arteries in healthy adults. Stroke. 1994;**25**:17-22

[41] Eliáš P, Žiška J. Dopplerovská ultrasonografie. Hradec Králové: Nucleus HK; 1998. p. 252

[42] Edvinson L, MacKenzie ET, McCullough J. Cerebral Blood Flow and Metabolism. New York: Raven Press; 1993. p. 683

[43] Faraci FM. Nitric oxide mediates vasodilatation in response to activation of N-methyl-D-aspartate receptors in brain. Circulation Research. 1993;**72**:476

[44] Wang WQ, Pelligrino DA, Baughman VL, Koenig HM, Albrecht RF. The role of neuronal nitric ixide synthase in regulation of cerebral blood flow in normocapnia and hypercapnia in rats. Journal of Cerebral Blood Flow and Metabolism. 1995;**15**: 774-778

[45] van Bel F, Valk L, Uiterwaal CSPM, Egberts J, Krediet TG. Plasma guanosine 3′5′cyclic monophosphate and severity of peri/intraventricular hemorrhage in the preterm newborn. Acta Paediatrica. 2002;**91**:434-439

[46] Lou YK, Wen C, Li M, Adams DJ, Wang MX, Yang F, et al. Decreased renal expression of nitric oxide synthase isoforms in adrenocorticotropin-induced and corticosteroid-induced hypertension. Hypertension. 2001;**37**: 1164-1170

[47] Crowley P. Prophylactic corticosteroids for preterm birth. In: Update Software,Issue 1 and Subseqeunt Issues. Oxford: The Cochrane Library; 1996

[48] Moise AA, Wearden ME, Kozinetz CA, Gest AL, Welty SE, Hansen TN. Antenatal steroids are associated with less need for blood pressure support in extremely premature infants. Paediatrics. 1995;**95**: 845-850

[49] Bonvento G, Seylaz J, Lacombe P. Widespread attenuation of cerebrovascular reactivity to hypercapnia following inhibition on nitric oxide synthase in the conscious rat. Journal of Cerebral Blood Flow and Metabolism. 1994;**14**:699

[50] Brian JE. Carbon dioxide and the cerebral ischemia. Anesthesiology. 1998; **88**:1365-1386

[51] Dreier JP, Körner K, Görner A, Lindauer U, Weih M, Villringer A, et al. Nitric oxide modulates the CBF response to increased extracellular potassium. Journal of Cerebral Blood Flow & Metabolism. 1995;**15**:914-919

[52] Kitazono T, Faraci FM, Taguchi H, Heistad DD. Role of potassium channels in cerebral blood vessels. Stroke. 1995; **26**:1713-1723

[53] Dirnagl U, Niwa K, Lindauer U, Villringer A. Coupling of cerebral blood flow to neuronal activation: Role of adenosine and nitric oxide. The American Journal of Physiology. 1994; **267**:296

[54] Sakabe T, Siesjö BK. The effect of indomethacin on the blood-flow-metabolism couple in the brain under normal, hypercapnic and hypoxic conditions. Acta Physiologica Scandinavica. 1979;**107**:283-284

[55] Mascia L, Fedorko L, Stewart DJ, Mohamed F, terBrugge K, Ranieri VM, et al. Temporal relationship between endothelin-1 concentrations and cerebral vasospasm in patients with aneurysmal subarachnoid hemorrhage. Stroke. 2001;**32**:1185-1190

[56] Nilsson T, Cantera L, Adner M, Edvinsson L. Presence of contractile endothelin-A and dilatory endothelin-B receptors in human cerebral arteries. Neurosurgery. 1997;**40**:346-351

[57] Harper AM, Glass HI. Effect of alterations in the arterial carbon dioxide tension on the blood flow through the cerebral cortex at normal and low arterial pressures. Journal of Neurology, Neurosurgery, and Psychiatry. 1965;**28**: 449-452

[58] Minárik M. Transkraniálna Farebná Duplexná Sonografia Dojčiat. Martin: Osveta; 2000. p. 148

[59] Gulbenkian S, Uddman R, Edvinson L. Neuronal messengers in the human cerebral circulation. Peptides. 2001;**22**:995-1007

[60] Morita-Tsuzuki Y, Hardebo JE, Bouskela E. Interaction between cerebrovascular sympathetic, parasympathetic and sensory nerves in blood flow regulation. Journal of Vascular Research. 1993;**30**:263-271

[61] Morita Y, Hardebo JE, Bouskela E. Influence of cerebrovascular sympathetic, parasympathetic, and sensory nerves on autoregulation and spontaneous vasomotion. Acta Physiologica Scandinavica. 1995;**154**: 121-130

[62] Bondar RL, Kassam MS, Stein F, Dunphy PT, Fortney S, Riedesel ML. Simultaneous cerebrovascular and cardiovascular responses during presyncope. Stroke. 1995;**26**:1794-1800

[63] Levine BD, Giller CA, Lane LD, Buckey JC, Blomqvist CG. Cerebral versus systemic hemodynamics during graded orthostatic stress in humans. Circulation. 1994;**90**:298-306

[64] Panerai RB. Assesment of cerebral pressure autoregulation in humans: A review of measurement methods. Physiological Measurement. 1998;**19**: 305-338

[65] Zhang R, Zuckerman JH, Levine BD. Deterioration of cerebral autoregulation during orthostatic stress: Insights from the frequency domain. Journal of Applied Physiology. 1998;**85**: 1113-1122

[66] Zhang R, Zuckerman JH, Iwasaki K, Wilson TE, Crandall CG, Levine BD. Autonomic neurol control of dynamic cerebral autoregulation in humans. Circulation. 2002;**106**:1814-1820

[67] Paulson OB, Strandgaard S, Edvinsson L. Cerebral autoregulation. Cerebrovascular and Brain Metabolism Reviews. 1990;**2**:161-192

[68] Sandor P. Nervous control of the cerebrovascular system: Doubts and facts. Neurochemistry International. 1999;**35**:237-259

[69] Lassen NA. Cerebral blood flow and oxygen consumption in man. Physiological review. American Journal of Physiology. 1959;**39**:183-238

[70] Ekström-Jodal B, Häggendal E, Linder LE. Cerebral blood flow autoregulation at high arterial pressures and different levels of carbon dioxide tension. European Neurology. 1972;**6**: 6-10

[71] Miller JD, Stanek AE, Langfitt TW. Cerebral blood flow regulation during experimental brain compression. Journal of Neurosurgery. 1973;**39**: 186-196

[72] Rasulo FA, Balestreri M, Matta B. Assessment of cerebral pressure autoregulation. Current Opinion in Anaesthesiology. 2002;**15**:483-488

[73] Panerai RB, Dawson SL, Eames PJ, Potter JF. Cerebral blood flow velocity response to induced and spontaneous sudden changes in arterial blood pressure. American Journal of Physiology. Heart and Circulatory Physiology. 2001;**280**:2162-2174

[74] Strebel S, Lam AM, Matta B, Mayberg TS, Aaslid R, Newell DW. Dynamic and static cerebral autoregulation during isoflurane, desflurane, and propofol anesthesia. Anesthesiology. 1995;**83**:66-76

[75] Powers WJ, Zazulia AR, Videen TO, Adams RE, Yundt KD, Aiyagari V, et al. Autoregulation of cerebral blood flow surrounding acute (6 to 22 hours) intracerebral hemorrhage. Neurology. 2001;**57**:18-24

[76] Traon AP, Costes-Salon MC, Galinier M, Fourcade J, Larrue V. Dynamic of cerebral blood flow autoregulation in hypertensive patients. Journal of the Neurological Sciences. 2002;**195**:139-144

[77] Harrison JM, Girling KJ, Mahajan RP. Effects of propofol and nitrous oxide on middle cerebral artery flow velocity and cerebral autoregulation. Anaesthesia. 2002;**57**: 27-32

[78] Summors A, Gupta A, Matta BF. Dynamic cerebral autoregulation during sevoflurane anaesthesia: A comparison with isoflurane. Anesthesia and Analgesia. 1999;**88**:341-345

[79] Tibble RK, Girling KJ, Mahajan RP. A comparison of transient hyperemic response test and static autoregulation tests to assess graded impairment in cerebral autoregulation during propofol, desflurane, and nitrous oxide anesthesia. Anesthésie et Analgésie. 2001;**93**:171-176

[80] Czosnyka M, Smielewski P. Monitoring of cerebral autoregulation in head-injured patients. Stroke. 1996;**27**: 1829-1834

[81] Czosnyka M, Smielewski P, Piechnik S, Steiner LA, Pickard JD. Cerebral autoregulation following head injury. Journal of Neurosurgery. 2001; **95**:756-763

[82] Juul N, Morris GF, Marshall SB, Marshall LF. Intracranial hypertension and cerebral perfusion pressure: Influence on neurological deterioration and outcome in severe head injury. The executive commitee of international selfotel trial. Journal of Neurosurgery. 2000;**92**:1-6

[83] Lam JMK, Smielevki P, Czosnyka M, Pickard JD, Kirkpatrick PJ. Predicting delayed ischemic deficits after subarachnoid hemorrhage using transient hyperemic response test of cerebral autoregulation. Neurosurgery. 2000;**47**:819-826

[84] Lang EW, Diehl RR, Mehdorn HM. Cerebral autoregulation testing after subarachnoid hemorrhage: The phase relationship between arterial blood pressure and cerebral blood flow

velocity. Critical Care Medicine. 2001; **29**:158-163

[85] Rapset T, Asser T. Cerebral hemodynamic impairment after aneurysmal subarachnoid hemorrhage as evaluated using transcranial doppler ultrasonography: Relationship to delayed cerebral ischemia and clinical outcome. Journal of Neurosurgery. 2001;**95**:393-401

[86] Lang EW, Chesnut RM. A bedside method for investigating the integrity and critical thresholds of cerebral pressure autoregulation in severe traumatic brain injury patients. British Journal of Neurosurgery. 2000;**14**: 117-126

[87] Steiner LA, Czosnyka M, Piechnik SK, Smielewski P, Chatfield D, Menon DK, et al. Continuous monitoring of cerebrovascular pressure reactivity allows determination of optimal cerebral perfusion pressure in patients with traumatic brain injury. Critical Care Medicine. 2002;**30**:733-738

[88] Greisen G. Cerebral blood flow in preterm infants during the first week of life. Acta Paediatrica Scandinavica. 1986;**75**:43-51

[89] Altman DI, Perlman JM, Volpe JJ, Powers WJ. Cerebral oxygen metabolism in newborns. Pediatrics. 1993;**92**:99-104

[90] Patel J, Marks K, Roberts I, Azzopardi D, Edwards AD. Measurement of cerebral blood flow in newborn infants using near infrared spectroscopy with indocyanine green. Pediatric Research. 1998;**43**:34-39

[91] Venkatesh B, Shen O, Lipman J. Continuous measurement of cerebral blood flow velocity using transcranial Doppler reveals significant moment-to-moment variability of data in healthy volunteers and in patients with subarachnoid hemorrhage. Critical Care Medicine. 2002;**30**:563-569

[92] Anthony MY. Cerebral autoregulation in sick infants. Pediatric Research. 2000;**48**:3-5

[93] Bullock R, Chesnut RM, Clifton G, Ghajar J, Marion DW, Narayan RK, et al. Guidelines for the management of severe head injury, Brain Trauma Foundation. European Journal of Emergency Medicine. 1996;**3**:109-127

[94] Czosnyka M, Smielewski P, Kirkpatrick P, Laing RJ, Menon D, Pickard JD. Continuous assessment of the cerebral vasomotor reactivity in head injury. Neurosurgery. 1997;**41**: 11-17

[95] Kett-White R, Hutchinson PJ, Czosnyka M. Multimodal monitoring of acute brain injury. Advances and Technical Standards in Neurosurgery. 2002;**27**:87-134

[96] Lang EW, Mehdom HM, Dorsch NWC. Continuous monitoring of cerebrovascular autoregulation: A validation study. Journal of Neurology, Neurosurgery, and Psychiatry. 2002;**72**: 583-586

[97] Nagai H, Moritake K, Takaya M. Correlation between transcranial Doppler ultrasonographic regional cerebral blood flow in experimental intracranial hypertension. Stroke. 1997; **28**:603-607

[98] Panerai RB. Transcranial Doppler for evaluation of cerebral autoregulation. Clinical Autonomic Research. 2009;**19**:197-211

[99] Rosner MJ, Rosner SD, Johnson AH. Cerebral perfusion pressure: Management protocol and clinical results. Journal of Neurosurgery. 1995; **83**:949-962

[100] Czosnyka M, Pickard J. The hyperaemic response to transient reduction in cerebral perfusion pressure:

A modeling study. Acta Neurochirurgica (Wien). 1992;**115**:90-97

[101] Panerai RB, Hudson V, Fan L, Mahony P, Yeoman PM, Hope T, et al. Assessment of dynamic autoregulation based on spontaneous fluctuations in arterial blood pressure and intracranial pressure. Physiological Measurement. 2002;**23**:59-72

[102] Rosengarten B, Kaps M. Peak systolic velocity doppler index reflects most appropriately the dynamic time course of intact cerebral autoregulation. Cerebrovascular Diseases. 2002;**13**: 230-234

[103] Smielewski P, Czosnyka M. Assessment of cerebral autoregulation using carotid artery compression. Stroke. 1996;**27**:2197-2203

[104] Steinmeier R, Bauhuf C. Slow rhythmic oscillations of blood pressure, intracranial pressure, microcirculation, and cerebral oxygenation. Stroke. 1996; **27**:2236-2243

[105] Tiecks F, Lam AM. Comparison of static and dynamic autoregulation measurements. Stroke. 1995;**26**: 1014-1019

[106] Aaslid R, Lindegaard KF, Sorteberg W, Nornes H. Cerebral autoregulation dynamics in humans. Stroke. 1989;**20**:45-52

[107] Dawson SL, Panerai RB. Dynamic but not static cerebral autoregulation is impaired in acute ischemic stroke. Cerebrovascular Diseases. 2000;**10**: 126-132

[108] Joó JG, Tóth Z, Beke A, Papp C, Tóth-Pál E, Csaba A, et al. Etiology, prenatal diagnostics and outcome of ventriculomegaly in 230 cases. Fetal Diagnosis and Therapy. 2008;**24**: 254-263

[109] Boylan GB, Young K, Panerai RB, Rennie JM, Evans DH. Dynamic cerebral autoregulation in sick newborn infants. Pediatric Research. 2000;**48**: 12-17

[110] Lou HC, Lassen NA, Friis-Hansen B. Impaired autoregulation of cerebral blood flow in the distressed newborn infants. The Journal of Pediatrics. 1979; **94**:118-121

[111] Panerai RB, Kelsall AWR, Rennie JM, Evans DH. Cerebral autoregulation dynamics in premature newborn. Stroke. 1995;**26**:74-80

[112] Jayasinghe D, Gill AB, Levene MI. CBF reactivity in hypotensive and normotensive preterm infants. Pediatric Research. 2003;**54**:848-853

[113] Tyszczuk L, Meek J, Elwell C, Wyatt JS. Cerebral blood flow is independent of mean arterial blood pressure in preterm infants undergoing intensive care. Pediatrics. 1998;**102**: 337-341

[114] Schmidek HH, Auer LM, Kapp JP. The cerebral venous system. Neurosurgery. 1985;**17**:663-678

[115] Varsík P, Kukumberg P. In: Varsik P et al., editors. Porucha pasáže v likvorových cestách a bolesti hlavy, Neurológia II, Patogenéza a klinika nervových chorôb. Bratislava: Lufema; 1999. pp. 398-402

[116] Barlow CF. CSF dynamics in hydrocephalus—with special attention to external hydrocephalus. Brain Dev. 1984;**6**:119-127

[117] Dickerman RB, McConathy WJ, Lustrin E, Schneider SJ. Rapid neurological deterioration associated with minor head trauma in chronic hydrocephalus. Child's Nervous System. 2003;**19**:249-251

[118] Šulla I. Arnoldova-Chiariho malformácia. In: Černý J et al., editors. Špeciálna chirurgia, Chirurgia krku a

hlavy. Vol. 4. Martin: Osveta; 1995. pp. 161-162

[119] Šulla I. Dandy-Walkerova malformácia. In: Černý J et al., editors. Špeciálna chirurgia, Chirurgia krku a hlavy. Vol. 4. Martin: Osveta; 1995. p. 167

[120] Casey AT, Kimmings EJ, Kleinlugtebeld AD, Taylor WA, Harkness WF, Hayward RD. The long-term outlook for hydrocephalus in childhood. Pediatric Neurosurgery. 1997;**27**:63-70

[121] Del Bigio MR. Future directions for therapy of childhood hydrocephalus: A view from the laboratory. Pediatric Neurosurgery. 2001;**34**:172-181

[122] Greitz D, Greitz T, Hindmarsh T. A new view on the CSF-circulation with the potential for pharmacological treatment of childhood hydrocephalus. Acta Paediatrica. 1997;**86**:125-132

[123] Hirsch JF. Consensus statement. Long term outcome in hydrocephalus. Child's Nervous System. 1994;**10**:64-69

[124] Hoppe-Hirsch E, Laroussine F, Brunet I, Sainte-Rose C, Renier D, Cinalli G, et al. Late outcome of the surgical treatment of hydrocephalus. Child's Nervous System. 1998;**14**:97-99

[125] McAllister JP, Chovan P. Neonatal hydrocephalus. Mechanism and consequences. Neurosurgery Clinics of North America. 1998;**9**:73-93

[126] Frim DM, Goumnerova LC. In vivo intracranial pressure dynamics in patients with hydrocephalus treated by shunt placement. Journal of Neurosurgery. 2000;**92**:927-932

[127] Tenti G, Drake JM, Sivaloganathan S. Brain biomechanics: Mathematical modeling of hydrocephalus. Neurological Research. 2000;**22**:19-24

[128] Tamaki N, Nagashima T, Ehara K, Kimura M, Matsumoto S, Iriguchi N. Changes in free water content and energy metabolism of the brain in experimental hydrocephalus. Acta Neurochirurgica. Supplement. 1990;**51**: 354-356

[129] Levine DN. Intracranial pressure and ventricular expansion in hydrocephalus: Have we been asking the wrong question? Journal of the Neurological Sciences. 2008;**269**:1-11

[130] Linninger AA, Sweetman B, Penn R. Normal and hydrocephalic brain dynamics: The role of reduced cerebrospinal fluid reabsorption in ventricular enlargement. Annals of Biomedical Engineering. 2009;**37**: 1434-1447

[131] Shulyakov AV, Buist RJ, Del Bigio MR. Intracranial biomechanics of acute experimental hydrocephalus in live rats. Neurosurgery. 2012;**71**: 1032-1040

[132] Klarica M, Oresković D, Bozić B, Vukić M, Butković V, Bulat M. New experimental model of acute aqueductal blockage in cats: Effects on cerebrospinal fluid pressure and the size of brain ventricles. Neuroscience. 2009; **158**:1397-1405

[133] Peña A, Bolton MD, Whitehouse H, Pickard JD. Effects of brain ventricular shape on periventricular biomechanics: A finite-element analysis. Neurosurgery. 1999;**45**:107-116

[134] Egnor M, Zheng L, Rosiello A, Gutman F, Davis R. A model of pulsations in communicating hydrocephalus. Pediatric Neurosurgery. 2002;**36**:281-303

[135] Matsushima T. Choroid plexus papillomas and human choroid plexus: A light and electron microscopic study. Journal of Neurosurgery. 1983;**59**: 1054-1062

[136] Welch K, Strand R, Bresnan M, Cavazzuti V. Congenital hydrocephalus due to villous hypertrophy of the telencephalic choroid plexuses: Case report. Journal of Neurosurgery. 1983; **59**:172-175

[137] Rekate HL. Classification of slit-ventricle syndromes using intracranial pressure monitoring. Pediatric Neurosurgery. 1993;**19**:15-20

[138] Rosman NP, Shands KN. Hydrocephalus caused by increased intracranial venous pressure: A clinicopathological study. Annals of Neurology. 1978;**3**:445-450

[139] Jones HC, Harris NG, Rocca JR, Andersohn RW. Progressive tissue injury in infantile hydrocephalus and prevention/reversal with shunt treatment. Neurological Research. 2000; **22**:89-96

[140] Takei F, Hirano A, Shapiro K, Kohn IJ. New ultrastructural changes of the ependyma in experimental hydrocephalus. Acta Neuropathologica. 1987;**73**:400-402

[141] Nakamura Y, Sato K. Role of disturbance of ependymal ciliary movement in development of hydrocephalus in rats. Child's Nervous System. 1993;**9**:65-71

[142] Castejon OJ. Transmission electron microscope study of human hydrocephalic cerebral cortex. Journal of Submicroscopic Cytology and Pathology. 1994;**26**:29

[143] Del Bigio MR, Bruni JE, Fewer HD. Human neonatal hydrocephalus: An electron microscopic study of the periventricular tissue. Journal of Neurosurgery. 1985;**63**:56-63

[144] Del Bigio MR. Neuropathological changes caused by hydrocephalus. Acta Neuropathologica. 1993;**85**:573-585

[145] Yamada H, Yokota A, Furuta A, Horie A. Reconstitution of shunted mantle in experimental hydrocephalus. Journal of Neurosurgery. 1992;**76**: 856-862

[146] Kriebel RM, Shah AB, McAllister JP 2nd. The microstructure of cortical neuropil before and after decompression in experimental infantile hydrocephalus. Experimental Neurology. 1993;**119**:89-98

[147] McAllister JP 2nd, Cohen MI, O'Mara KA, Johnson MH. Progression of experimental infantile hydrocephalus and effects of ventriculoperitoneal shunts: An analysis correlatim magmetic resonance imaging with gross morphology. Neurosurgery. 1991;**29**: 329-340

[148] Azzi GM, Canady AI, Ham S, Mitchell JA. Kaolin-induced hydrocephalus in the hamster: Temporal sequence of changes in intracranial pressure, ventriculomegaly and whole-brain specific gravity. Acta Neuropathologica. 1999;**98**:245-250

[149] Tamaki N, Yamashita H, Kimura M, Ehara K, Asada M, Nagashima T, et al. Changes in the components and content of biological water in the brain of experimental rabbits. Journal of Neurosurgery. 1990; **73**:274-278

[150] Tamaki N, Yamashita H, Kimura M, Ehara K, Asada M, Nagashima T, et al. Changes in the components and content of biological water in the brain of experimental hydrocephalic rabbits. Journal of Neurosurgery. 1990;**73**:274-278

[151] Talman WT, Florek G, Bullard DE. A hyperthermic syndrome in two subjects with acute hydrocephalus. Archives of Neurology. 1988;**45**: 1037-1040

[152] Robles P, Poblano A, Hernandez G, Ibarra J, Guzman I, Sosa J. Cortical, brainstem and autonomic nervous system dysfunction in infants with post-hemorrhagic hydrocephalus. Revista de Investigación Clínica. 2002;**54**:133-138

[153] Uhríková Z, Kolarovszki B, Javorka K, Javorka M, Maťašová K, Kolarovszká H, et al. Changes in heart rate variability in a premature infant with hydrocephalus. American Journal of Perinatology Reports. 2012;**2**:43-46

[154] Oka N, Nakada J, Endo S, Takaku A. Angioarchitecture in experimental hydrocephalus. Pediatric Neuroscience. 1986;**12**:294-299

[155] Oka N, Nakada J, Nagahori T, Erdo S, Takaku A. Changes in the cerebral vascular bed in experimental hydrocephalus: An angioarchitectural and histological study. In: Matsumoto S, Tamaki N, editors. Hydrocephalus-pathogenesis and Treatment. Tokyo: Springer-Verlag; 1991. pp. 46-57

[156] Okuyama T, Hashi K, Sasaki S, Sudo K, Kurokawa Y. Changes in cerebral microvasculature in congenital hydrocephalus of the inbred rat LEW/Jms: Light and electron microscopic examination. Surgical Neurology. 1987; **27**:338-342

[157] Ransohoff J, Dimattio J, Hochwald G, Epstein F. Cerebral fluid dynamics and brain regional blood flow in experimental hydrocephalus. Child's Brain. 1975;**1**:183-186

[158] Sato O, Ohya M, Nojiri K, Tsugane R. Microcirculatory changes in experimental hydrocephalus: Morphological and physiological studies. In: Shapiro K, Marmarou A, Portnoy H, editors. Hydrocephalus. New York: Raven Press; 1984. pp. 215-230

[159] Luciano MG, Skarupa DJ, Booth AM, Wood AS, Brant CL, Gdowski MJ. Cerebrovascular adaptation in chronic hydrocephalus. Journal of Cerebral Blood Flow and Metabolism. 2001;**21**:285-294

[160] Del Bigio MR, Massicotte EM. Protective effect of nimodipine on behavior and white matter of rats with hydrocephalus. Journal of Neurosurgery. 2001;**94**:788-794

[161] da Silva MC, Michowicz S, Drake JM, Chumas PD, Tuor UI. Reduced local cerebral blood flow in periventricular white matter in experimental neonatal hydrocephalus—restoration with CSF shunting. Journal of Cerebral Blood Flow and Metabolism. 1995;**15**:1057-1065

[162] Bateman GA. Vascular compliance in normal pressure hydrocephalus. American Journal of Neuroradiology. 2000;**21**:1574-1585

[163] Bradley WG. Normal pressure hydrocephalus and deep white matter ischemia: Which is the chicken, and which is the egg? American Journal of Neuroradiology. 2001;**22**:1638-1640

[164] Owler BK, Pickard JD. Normal pressure hydrocephalus and cerebral blood flow: A review. Acta Neurologica Scandinavica. 2001;**104**:325-342

[165] Cerda M, Vielma J, Martinez C, Basauri L. Poly-acrylamide gel electrophoresis of cerebrospinal fluid proteins in children with nontumoral hydrocephalus. Child's Brain. 1980;**6**: 140-149

[166] Chumas PD, Drake JM, Del Bigio MR, Da Silva M, Tuor UI. Anaerobic glycolysis preceding white-matter destruction in experimental neonatal hydrocephalus. Journal of Neurosurgery. 1994;**80**:491-501

[167] Kizu O, Yamada K, Nishimura T. Proton chemical shift imaging in normal pressure hydrocephalus. American

Journal of Neuroradiology. 2001;**22**: 1659-1664

[168] Nussinovitch M, Volovitz B, Finkelstein Y, Amir J, Harel D. Lactic dehydrogenase isoenzymes in cerebrospinal fluid associated with hydrocephalus. Acta Paediatrica. 2001; **90**:972-974

[169] Onodera Y, Kawaguchi T, Itoh H. Fatty acid of cerebrospinal fluid in arrested hydrocephalus. Child's Brain. 1982;**9**:95-101

[170] Ding Y, McAllister JP 2nd, Yao B, Yan N, Canady AI. Neuron tolerance during hydrocephalus. Neuroscience. 2001;**106**:659-667

[171] Shinoda M, Hidaka M, Lindquist E, Soderstrom S, Matsumae M, Sato O, et al. NGF, NT-3 and Trk C mRNA, but not Trk A mRNA, are upregulated in the paraventricular structures in experimental hydrocephalus. Child's Nervous System. 2001;**17**:704-712

[172] Del Bigio MR. Calcium-mediated proteolytic damage in white matter of hydrocephalic rats? Journal of Neuropathology and Experimental Neurology. 2000;**59**:946-954

[173] Caner H, Atasever A, Kilinc K, Durgun B, Peker S, Ozcan OE. Lipid peroxide level increase in experimental hydrocephalus. Acta Neurochirurgica. 1993;**121**:68-71

[174] Tashiro Y, Drake JM, Chakrabortty S, Hattori T. Functional injury of cholinergic, GABAergic and dopaminergic systems in the basal ganglia of adult rat with kaolin-induced hydrocephalus. Brain Research. 1997; **770**:45-52

[175] Chovanes GI, McAllister JP 2nd, Lamperti AA, Salotto AG, Truex RC Jr. Monoamine alterations during experimental hydrocephalus in neonatal rats. Neurosurgery. 1988;**22**:86-91

[176] Zhang YW, Del Bigio MR. Growth-associated protein-43 is increased in cerebrum of immature rats following induction of hydrocephalus. Neuroscience. 1998;**86**:847-854

[177] Suda K, Sato K, Miyazawa T, Arai H. Changes of synapse-related proteins (SVP-38 and drebrins) during development of brain in congenitally hydrocephalic HTX rats with and without early placement of ventriculoperitoneal shunt. Pediatric Neurosurgery. 1994;**20**:50-56

[178] Masago A, Shimada S, Minami Y, Inoue K, Morimura H, Otori Y, et al. GLAST mRNA expression in the periventricular area of experimental hydrocephalus. Neuroreport. 1996;**7**: 2565-2570

[179] Koehne P, Hochhaus F, Felderhoff-Muesser U, Ring-Mrozik E, Obladen M, Buhrer C. Vascular endothelial growth factor and erythropoietin concentrations in cerebrospinal fluid of children with hydrocephalus. Child's Nervous System. 2002;**18**:137-141

[180] Tamaki N, Yasuda M, Matsumoto S, Yamamoto T, Iriguchi N. Cerebral energy metabolism in experimental canine hydrocephalus. Child's Nervous System. 1990;**6**:172-178

[181] da Silva MC, Drake JM, Lemaire C, Cross A, Tuor UI. High-energy phosphate metabolism in a neonatal model of hydrocephalus before and after shunting. Journal of Neurosurgery. 1994;**81**:544-553

[182] Braun KP, van Eijsden P, Vandertop WP, de Graaf RA, Gooskens RH, Tulleken KA, et al. Cerebral metabolism in experimental hydrocephalus: An in vivo 1H and 31P magnetic resonance spectroscopy study. Journal of Neurosurgery. 1999;**91**: 660-668

[183] Harris NG, Plant HD, Inglis BA, Briggs RW, Jones HC. Neurochemical

changes in the cerebral cortex of treated and untreated hydrocephalic rat pups quantified with in vitro 1H-NMR spectroscopy. Journal of Neurochemistry. 1997;**68**:305-312

[184] Kolarovszki B, De Riggo J. Biomechanika a monitoring vnútrolebkovej dynamiky u novorodencov a detí s hydrocefalom. Praktická Medicína. 2008;**2**:16-18

[185] Kolarovszki B, De Riggo J, Ďurdík P, Maťašová K, Kolarovszká H, Benčo M. Detský hydrocefalus. Neurológia. 2009;**4**:13-17

[186] Kolarovszki B, De Riggo J, Ďurdík P, Kolarovszká H, Benčo M. Manažment novorodeneckého a detského hydrocefalu. Neurológia. 2008;**3**:41-44

[187] Kolarovszki B, Kolarovszká H. Intrakraniálna dynamika novorodeneckého hydrocefalu. Pokroky v perinatológii: Zborník vedeckých prác CEPV. Martin: Jesseniova lekárska fakulta Univerzity Komenského v Martine a CA KAMI; 2011. pp. 95-100

[188] Kolarovszki B, Benčo M, Ďurdík P, Murgaš D, Hanula M, Kolarovszká H, et al. Detský hydrocefalus ako akútny stav. In: Hanula M, Murgaš D, Csomor D, editors. Vybrané kapitoly z urgentnej medicíny. Nitra: Inštitút zdravotníckeho vzdelávania; 2009. pp. 198-202

[189] Kolarovszki B, De Riggo J, Ďurdík P, Šutovský J. Sledovanie intrakraniálnej dynamiky detského hydrocefalu. Pediatria. 2006;**1**:132-135

[190] Fenton TR. A new growth chart for preterm babies: Babson and Benda's chart updated with recent data and a new format. BMC Pediatrl; Dec 16 2003;**3**:13

[191] Kolarovszki B, De Riggo J, Ďurdík P, Šutovský J, Kolarovszká H, Zubríková L, et al. Menežment dieťaťa s hydrocefalom. Diagnostika a terapia v pediatrii 9. Martin: Univerzita Komenského v Bratislave Jesseniova lekárska fakulta v Martine; 2007. pp. 82-84

[192] Di Rocco C, Caldarelli M, Ceddia A. "Occult" hydrocephalus in children. Child's Nervous System. 1989;**5**:71-75

[193] Hanlo PW, Gooskens RH, Faber JA, Peters RJ, Hermsen AA, Nijhuis IJ, et al. Relationship between anterior fontanel pressure measurements and clinical signs in infantile hydrocephalus. Child's Nervous System. 1996;**12**:200-209

[194] Kirkpatrick M, Engleman H, Minns RA. Symptoms and signs of progressive hydrocephalus. Archives of Disease in Childhood. 1989;**64**:124-128

[195] Kolarovszki B, De Riggo J. Hodnotenie klinických príznakov intrakraniálnej hypertenzie vo vzťahu k indikácii drenážneho výkonu u novorodencov a dojčiat s hydrocefalom. Česko-slovenská Pediatrie. 2008;**63**: 521-527

[196] Bech RA, Juhler M. Unusual clinical manifestations of disturbed CSF dynamics in hydrocephalic children. Child's Nervous System. 2000;**16**: 446-450

[197] Eide PK, Due-Tønnessen B, Helseth E, Lundar T. Differences in quantitative characteristics of intracranial pressure in hydrocephalic children treated surgically or conservatively. Pediatric Neurosurgery. 2002;**36**:304-313

[198] Eide PK, Fremming AD. A new method and software for quantitative analysis of continuous intracranial pressure recordings. Acta Neurochirurgica. 2001;**143**:1237-1247

[199] Foyas IP, Casey ATH, Thompson D, Harkness WF, Hayward RD. Use of intracranial

pressure monitoring in the management of childhood hydrocephalus and shunt-related problems. Neurosurgery. 1996; **38**:726-732

[200] Walsh P, Logan WJ. Continuous and intermittent measurement of intracranial pressure by Ladd monitor. The Journal of Pediatrics. 1983;**102**: 439-442

[201] Easa D, Tran A, Bingham W. Noninvasive intracranial pressure measurement in the newborn. American Journal of Diseases of Children. 1983; **137**:332-335

[202] Bass JK, Bass WT, Green GA, Gurtner P, White LE. Intracranial pressure changes during intermittent CSF drainage. Pediatric Neurology. 2003;**28**:173-177

[203] Sainte-Rose C, Piatt JH, Renier D, Pierre-Kahn A, Hirsch JF, Hoffman HJ, et al. Mechanical complications in shunts. Pediatric Neurosurgery. 1991-1992;**17**:2-9

[204] Lazareff JA, Peacock W, Holly L, Ver Halen J, Wong A, Olmstead C. Multiple shunt failure: An analysis of relevant factors. Child's Nervous System. 1998;**14**:271-275

[205] Collins P, Hockley AD, Woolam DHM. Surface ultrastructure of tissues occluding ventricular catheters. Journal of Neurosurgery. 1978;**48**: 609-613

[206] Drake JM, Kestle JRW, Milner R, Cinalli G, Boop F, Piatt J, et al. Randomised trial of cerebrospinal fluid shunt valve design in paediatric hydrocephalus. Neurosurgery. 1998;**43**: 294-305

[207] Porter RW, Detwiler PW, Rekate HL. Hydrocephalus in children. In: Kaye AH, Black PML, editors. Operative Neurosurgery. London: Churchill Livingstone; 2000. pp. 1215-1233

[208] Kolarovszki B, Šutovský J, De Riggo J, Ďurdík P, Kolarovszká H. Možnosti operačnej liečby detského hydrocefalu. Pediatria. 2006;**1**:281-284

[209] Nosáľ S, Čiljak M, Šutovský J, Kolarovszki B, Ľuptáková A. Hydrocefalus—komplikácie ventrikuloperitoneálneho shuntu. Diagnostika a terapia v pediatrii. Martin: Jesseniova lekárska fakulta UK; 2004. pp. 115-119

[210] Lipina R, Paleček T. Chirurgická léčba hydrocefalu v dětském věku. Pediatrie pro praxi. 2004;**3**:133-136

[211] Novák Z, Chrastina J. Neuroendoskopie. Praha: Maxdorf s.r.o; 2005. p. 138

[212] Jones RFC, Kwok BCT, Stening WA, Vonau M. Neuroendoscopic third ventriculostomy: A practical alternative to extracranial shunts in non-communicating hydrocephalus. Acta Neurochirurgica. 1994;**61**(suppl):79-83

[213] Sainte-Rose C, Chumas P. Endoscopic third ventriculostomy. Techniques in Neurosurgery. 1996;**1**: 176-184

[214] Brockmeyer D, Abtin K, Carey L, Walker M. Endoscopic third ventriculostomy: An outcome analysis. Pediatric Neurosurgery. 1998;**28**: 236-240

[215] Goumnerova LC, Frim DM. Treatment of hydrocephalus with third ventriculostomy outcome and CSF flow patterns. Pediatric Neurosurgery. 1997; **27**:149-152

[216] Teo C. Jones R, Management of hydrocephalus by endoscopic third ventriculostomy in patients with myelomeningocele. Pediatric Neurosurgery. 1996;**25**:57-63

[217] Tuli S, Ashail E, Drake J. Third ventriculostomy versus cerebrospinal

fluid shunt as a first procedure in pediatric hydrocephalus. Pediatric Neurosurgery. 1999;**30**:11-15

[218] Vinchon M, Rekate H, Kulkarni AV. Pediatric hydrocephalus outcomes: A review. Fluids and Barriers of the CNS. 2012;**9**:18

[219] Warf BC, Tracy S, Mugamba J. Long-term outcome for endoscopic third ventriculostomy alone or in combination with choroid plexus cauterization for congenital aqueductal stenosis in African infants. Journal of Neurosurgery. Pediatrics. 2012;**10**: 108-111

[220] Scarrow AM, Levy EI, Pascucci L, Albright AL. Outcome analysis of endoscopic III ventriculostomy. Child's Nervous System. 2000;**16**:442-445

[221] Siomin V, Cinalli G, Grotenhuis A, Golash A, Oi S, Kothbauer K, et al. Endoscopic third ventriculostomy in patients with cerebrospinal fluid infection and/or hemorrhage. Journal of Neurosurgery. 2002;**97**:519-524

[222] Yadav YR, Jaiswal S, Adam N, Basoor A, Jain G. Endoscopic third ventriculostomy in infants. Neurology India. 2006;**54**:161-163

[223] Costa Val JA, Scaldaferri PM, Furtado LM, de Souza Baptista G. Third ventriculostomy in infants younger than 1 year old. Child's Nervous System. 2012;**28**:1233-1235

[224] Engel M, Carmel PW, Chutorian AM. Increased intraventricular pressure without ventriculomegaly in children with shunts: "normal volume" hydrocephalus. Neurosurgery. 1979;**5**: 549-552

[225] Leggate JRS, Baxter P, Minns RA, Steers AJWS, Brown JK, Shaw JF, et al. Role of a separeted subcutaneous cerebro-spinal fluid reservoir in the management of hydrocephalus. British Journal of Neurosurgery. 1988;**2**:327-337

[226] Gilkes CE, Steers AJW, Minns RA. Pressure compensation in shunt-dependent hydrocephalus with CSF shunt malfunction. Child's Nervous System. 2001;**17**:52-57

[227] Katz DM, Trobe JD, Muraszko KM, Dauser RC. Shunt failure without ventriculomegaly proclaimed by ophtalmic findings. Journal of Neurosurgery. 1994;**81**:721-725

[228] Kölfen W, Korinthenberg R, Schmidt H. Bedrohliche Hirndruckkrisen bei draniertem Hydrocephalus mit minimal erweiterten oder normalen Ventrikeln. Monatsschrift für Kinderheilkunde. 1989;**137**:297-301

[229] Lee TT, Uribe J, Ragheb J, Morrison G, Jagid JR. Unique clinical presentation of pediatric shunt malfunction. Pediatric Neurosurgery. 1999;**30**:122-126

[230] McCullough DC, Balzer-Martin LA. Current prognosis in overt neonatal hydrocephalus. Journal of Neurosurgery. 1982;**57**:378-383

[231] Renier D, Sainte-Rose C, Pierre-Kahn A, et al. Prenatal hydrocephalus: Outcome and prognosis. Child's Nervous System. 1988;**4**:213-222

[232] Barnes NP, Jones SJ, Hayward RD, Harkness WJ, Thompson D. Ventriculoperitoneal shunt block: What are the best predictive clinical indicators? Archives of Disease in Childhood. 2002;**87**:198-201

[233] Watkins L, Hayward R, Andar U, Harkness W. The diagnosis of blocked cerebrospinal fluid shunts: A prospective study of referral to a paediatric neurosurgical unit. Child's Nervous System. 1994;**10**:87-90

[234] Arnell K, Eriksson E, Olsen L. Asymptomatic shunt malfunction detected fortuitously by observation of papilloedema. Acta Neurochirurgica. 2003;**145**:1093-1096

[235] Constantini S, Umansky F, Nesher R, Shalit M. Transient blindness following intracranial pressure changes in a hydrocephalic child with a V-P shunt. Child's Nervous System. 1987;**3**: 379-381

[236] Available from: http://eyewiki.aao.org/Papilledema

[237] Arroyo HA, Jan JE, McCormick AQ, Farrell K. Permanent visual loss after shunt malfunction. Neurology. 1985;**35**:25-29

[238] Gaston H. Ophthalmic complications of spina bifida and hydrocephalus. Eye. 1991;**5**:279-290

[239] Chou SY, Digre KB. Neuro-ophthalmic complications of raised intracranial pressure, hydrocephalus, and shunt malfunction. Neurosurgery Clinics of North America. 1999;**10**: 587-608

[240] Nazir S, O'Brien M, Qureshi NH, Slape L, Green TJ, Phillips PH. Sensitivity of papilledema as a sign of shunt failure in children. Journal of AAPOS. 2009;**13**:63-66

[241] Kimmings E, Kleinugtebeld AD, Casey AT, Hayward RD. Does the child with shunted hydrocephalus require long-term neurosurgical follow-up? British Journal of Neurosurgery. 1996; **10**:77-81

[242] Kováč A. Abdominálna Ultrasonografia. Martin: Osveta; 1995. p. 384

[243] Taylor KJW, Holland S. Doppler US. Part I. Basis principles instrumentations, and pitfalls. Radiology. 1990;**174**:297-303

[244] Barnett SB, Ziskin MC, Ter Haar GR, Rott HD, Duck FA, Maeda K. International recommendations and guidelines for the safe use of diagnostic ultrasound. Ultrasound in Medicine & Biology. 2000;**26**:355-366

[245] Višňovský J. Vyšetrenie cirkulácie v pôrodníctve. Osveta: Martin; 2002. p. 200

[246] American Institute of Ultrasound in Medicine, Bioeffects Commitee. Bioeffects considerations for the safety of diagnostic ultrasound. Ultrasound in Medicine and Biology. 1988;**7**(suppl):S1-S38

[247] Doida Y. Confirmation of an ultrasound-induced mutation in two in-vitro mammalian cell lines. Ultrasound in Medicine & Biology. 1990;**16**:699-705

[248] Baggs R, Penney DP, Cox C, Child SZ. Threshold for ultrasonically-induced lung hemorrhage in neonatal swine. Ultrasound in Medicine & Biology. 1996;**22**:119-128

[249] Dalecki D, Child SZ, Raeman CH, Cox C, Carstensen EL. Ultrasonically-induced lung hemorrhage in young swine. Ultrasound in Medicine & Biology. 1997;**23**:177-181

[250] Frizzell LA, Chen E, Chong L. Effect of pulsed ultrasound on the mouse neonate: Hind limb paralysis and lung hemorrhage. Ultrasound in Medicine & Biology. 1994;**20**:53-63

[251] Holland CK, Zheng X, Apfel RE, Alderman JL, Fernandez L, Taylor KJW. Direct evidence of cavitation in vivo from diagnostic ultrasound. Ultrasound in Medicine & Biology. 1996;**22**:917-925

[252] Zacchary JG, O'Brien WD. Lung lesions induced by continuous and pulsed wave (diagnostic) ultrasound in mice, rabbits and pigs. Veterinary Pathology. 1995;**32**:43-54

[253] Duck FA. Acoustic streaming and radiation pressure in diagnostic application: What are the implication? In: Barrett SB, Kossoff G, editors. Safety of Diagnostic Ultrasound. Carnforth, UK: Pathenon Publishing; 1998. pp. 87-98

[254] Available from: http://www.rhythmodynamics.com/Gabriel_LaFreniere/sa_Doppler.htm

[255] Brenet O, Granry JC, Poirier N, Le Gall R. The effect of desflurane on cerebral blood flow velocity and cerebrovascular reactivity to CO_2 in children. Annales Françaises d'Anesthèsie et de Rèanimation. 1998;**17**: 227-233

[256] Zibolen M. Dopplerovská sonografia obličiek plodov, novorodencov a detí. Martin: Flipo s. r. o; 2000. p. 178

[257] Merritt CRB. Doppler color flow imaging. Journal of Clinical Ultrasound. 1987;**15**:591-597

[258] Fisher AQ, Aziz E, Blalock A. Color flow doppler sonography of intracranial arteries (abstract). Annals of Neurology. 1988;**24**:344

[259] Tatsuno M, Kubota T, Okuyama K, Kawauchi A. Intracranial vessels with color doppler echoencephalography in infants. Brain and Development. 1989;**2**: 125-130

[260] Wong TS, Tsuruda JS, Liberman RL, Chirino A, Vogt JF, Gangitano E. Color Doppler imaging of intracranial vessels in the neonate. AJR. 1989;**152**:1065-1070

[261] Mitchell DG, Merton DA, Needleman L, Kurtz AB, Goldberg BB, Levy D, et al. Neonatal brain: Color Doppler imaging, Part I. Technique and vascular anatomy. Radiology. 1988;**167**: 303-306

[262] Fox JL, Richards JR, Luessenhop AJ. Method for detecting intracranial arteriovenous malformation with an ultrasonic transducer using the Doppler phenomenon. Journal of Neurosurgery. 1967;**26**:322-326

[263] White DN. The early development of neurosonology: III. Pulsatile echoencephalography and Doppler techniques. Ultrasound in Medicine & Biology. 1992;**18**:323-376

[264] Bada HS, Hajjar W, Chua C, Summer DS. Noninvasive diagnosis of neonatal asphyxia and intraventricular hemorrhage by Doppler ultrasound. The Journal of Pediatrics. 1979;**95**:775-779

[265] Aaslid R, Markwalder TM, Nornes H. Noninvasive transcranial Doppler ultrasound recording of flow velocity in basal cerebral arteries. Journal of Neurosurgery. 1982;**57**: 769-774

[266] Kolarovszki B, De Riggo J, Ďurdík P, Maťašová K, Kolarovszká H, Zubríková L, et al. Využitie transkraniálnej dopplerovskej sonografie v manažmente novorodencov a dojčiat s hydrocefalom. Pediatria. 2007;**2**:325-328

[267] Available from: http://pmj.bmj.com/content/83/985/683.full

[268] De Oliveira RS, Machado HR. Transcranial color-coded Doppler ultrasonography for evaluation of children with hydrocephalus. Neurosurgical Focus. 2003;**15**:1-7

[269] Taylor GA, Madsen JR. Neonatal hydrocephalus: Hemodynamic response to fontanelle compression—Correlation with intracranial pressure and need for shunt placement. Radiology. 1996;**201**: 685-689

[270] Taylor GA, Phillips MD, Ichord RN, Carson BS, Gates JA, James CS. Intracranial compliance in

infants: Evaluation with Doppler US. Radiology. 1994;**191**:787-791

[271] Westra SJ, Lazareff J, Curran JG, Sayere JW, Kawamoto H Jr. Transcranial Doppler ultrasonography to evaluate need for cerebrospinal fluid drainage in hydrocephalic children. Journal of Ultrasound in Medicine. 1998; **17**:561-569

[272] Kirsch JR, Traystman RJ, Rogers MC. Cerebral blood flow measurement techniques in infants and children. Pediatrics. 1985;**75**:887-895

[273] Greisen G. Methods for assessing cerebral blood flow. In: Levene MI, Bennett MJ, Punt J, editors. Fetal and Neonatal Neurology and Neurosurgery. 1988. pp. 151-161

[274] Ruissen CJ, van Vugt JM, Hoogland HJ, Hoeks AP, de Haan J. Technical aspect of fetal doppler measurements. Gynecologic and Obstetric Investigation. 1987;**24**:1-13

[275] van de Bor M, Walther F, Simms ME. Acceleration time in cerebral arteries in preterm infants. Journal of Clinical Ultrasound. 1990;**18**: 267-271

[276] Aaslid R. Transcranial Doppler Ultrasonography. New York: Springer-Verlag; 1986. p. 482

[277] Arnolds BJ, von Reutern GM. Transcranial Doppler sonography: Examination technique and normal reference values. Ultrasound in Medicine & Biology. 1986;**115**:115-123

[278] Babikian VL, Wechsler LR. Transcranial Doppler Ultrasonography. St. Louis: Mosby-Year Book Inc.; 1993. p. 323

[279] Lindegaard KL. Variations in middle cerebral artery blood flow investigated with noninvasive transcranial blood flow velocity measurements. Stroke. 1987;**18**: 1025-1030

[280] von Reutern GM, Büdingen HJ. Ultraschalldiagnostik der hirnversorgenden Arterien. Stuttgart: Thieme-Verlag; 1988. p. 381

[281] Ringelstein EB, Kahlscheuer E, Niggemeyer E, Otis SM. Transcranial Doppler sonography: Anatomical landmarks and normal velocity values. Ultrasound in Medicine & Biology. 1990;**16**:745-761

[282] Sorteberg W. Side-to-side differences and day-to-day variations of transcranial Doppler parameters in normal subjects. Journal of Ultrasound in Medicine. 1990;**9**:403-409

[283] Deeg KK, Rupprecht TH. Pulsed Doppler sonographic measurement of normal values for the flow velocities in the intracranial arteries of healthy newborns. Pediatric Radiology. 1989;**19**: 71-78

[284] Bode H. Pediatric Applications of Transcranial Doppler Sonography. Vienna: Springer-Verlag; 1988. p. 326

[285] Hayashi T, Ichiyama T, Uchida M, Tashiro N, Tanaka H. Evaluation by colour Doppler and pulsed Doppler sonography of blood flow velocities in intracranial arteries during the early neonatal period. European Journal of Pediatrics. 1992;**151**:461-465

[286] Ozek E, Koroglu TF, Karakoc F. Transcranial Doppler assessment of cerebral blood flow velocity in term newborns. European Journal of Pediatrics. 1995;**154**:60-63

[287] Lin KL, Chen KS, Hsieh MY, Wang HS. Transcranial color Doppler sonography on healthy pre-school children: Flow velocities and total cerebral blood flow volume. Brain and Development. 2007;**29**:64-68

[288] Muniz IA, Netto AA, Gonçalves VM. Neonatal Doppler velocimetry in full term small-for-gestational age newborns. Arquivos de Neuro-Psiquiatria. 2003;**61**:808-815

[289] Kolarovszki B, Zibolen M. Transcranial doppler ultrasonography in the management of neonatal hydrocephalus. In: Pant S, Cherian I, editors. Hydrocephalus. Rijeka: InTech; 2012. pp. 131-152

[290] Menke J, Michel E, Rabe H, Bresser W, Grohs B, Schidtt M, et al. Simultaneous influence of blood flow pressure, pCO_2, pO_2 on cerebral blood flow velocity in preterm infants of less than 33 weeks gestation. Pediatric Research. 1993;**34**:173-177

[291] Miller JD, Smith RR, Holaday HR. Carbon dioxide reactivity in the evaluation of cerebral ischemia. Neurosurgery. 1992;**30**:518-521

[292] Bissonnette B, Benson LN. Closure of persistently patent arterial duct and its impact on cerebral circulatory haemodynamics in children. Canadian Journal of Anesthesia. 1998;**45**:199-205

[293] Jurko A Jr, Jurko A, Hlaučová E, Zibolen M, Šparcová A. Dynamika niektorých hemodynamických parametrov vo včasnom novorodeneckom období. Bratislavské Lekárske Listy. 1995;**96**:325-330

[294] Ausina A, Baquena M, Nadal M, Manrique S, Ferrer A, Sahuquillo J, et al. Cerebral haemodynamic changes during sustained hypocapnia in severe head injury: Can hyperventilation cause cerebral ischemia? Acta Neurochirurgica. Supplement. 1988;**71**: 1-4

[295] Curz J. The first decade of continuous monitoring of jugular bulb oxyhemoglobinsaturation: Management strategies and clinical outcome. Critical Care Medicine. 1998;**26**:344-351

[296] Levene MI. Cerebral blood flow. In: Levene M, editor. Neonatal Neurology. Churchill Livingstone; 1987. pp. 23-44

[297] Daven JR, Milstein JM, Guthrie RD. Cerebral vascular resistance in premature infant. American Journal of Diseases of Children. 1983;**137**:85-93

[298] Krcho P. Ultrazvukové vyšetrenie mozgu novorodenca. Lek Obz. 2005;**54**: 508-511

[299] Zibolen M, Zbojan J, Dluholucký S. Praktická neonatológia. Osveta: Martin; 2001. p. 534

[300] Antes S, Kiefer M, Schmitt M, Lechtenfeld M, Geipel M, Eymann R. Frontal and temporal horn ratio: A valid and reliable index to determine ventricular size in paediatric hydrocephalus patients? Acta Neurochirurgica. Supplement. 2012;**114**: 227-230

[301] Davies MW, Swaminathan M, Chuang SL, Betheras FR. Reference ranges for the linear dimensions of the intracranial ventricles in preterm neonates. Archives of Disease in Childhood. Fetal and Neonatal Edition. 2000;**82**:F218-F223

[302] Perry RNW, Bowman ED, Roy RND, de Crespigny LC. Ventricular size in newborn infants. Journal of Ultrasound in Medicine. 1985;**4**:475-477

[303] Monteagudo A, Haratz-Rubinstein N, Timor-Tritsch IE. Biometry of the fetal brain. In: Timor-Tritsch IE, Monteagudo A, Cohen HL, editors. Ultrasonography of the Prenatal and Neonatal Brain. Connecticut: Appleton and Lange; 1996. pp. 89-146

[304] Sauerbrei EE, Digney M, Harrison PB, Cooperberg PL. Ultrasonic evaluation of neonatal intra-cranial hemorrhage and its complications. Radiology. 1981;**139**:677-685

[305] Levene MI. Measurement of the growth of lateral ventricles in preterm infants with real-time ultrasound. Archives of Disease in Childhood. 1981; **56**:900-904

[306] Liao M, Chaou W, Tsao L, Nishida H, Sakanoue M. Ultrasound measurement of the ventricular size in newborn infants. Brain and Development. 1986;**8**:262-268

[307] Sondhi V, Gupta G, Gupta PK, Patnaik SK, Tshering K. Establishment of nomograms and reference ranges for intra-cranial ventricular dimensions and ventriculo-hemispheric ratio in newborns by ultrasonography. Acta Paediatrica. 2008;**97**:738-744

[308] Evans W. An encephalographic ratio for estimating ventricular enlargement and cerebral atrophy. Archives of Neurology and Psychiatry. 1942;**47**:931-937

[309] Kulkarni AV, Drake JM, Armstrong DC, Dirks PB. Measurement of ventricular size: Reliability of the frontal and occipital horn ratio compared to subjective assessment. Pediatric Neurosurgery. 1999;**31**:65-70

[310] Eide PK. The relationship between intracranial pressure and size of cerebral ventricles assessed by computed tomography. Acta Neurochirurgica. 2003;**145**:171-179

[311] Hanlo PW, Gooskens RJHM, van Schooneveld M, Tulleken CAF, van der Knaap MS, Faber JAJ, et al. The effect of intracranial pressure on myelination and the relationship with neurodevelopment in infantile hydrocephalus. Developmental Medicine and Child Neurology. 1997;**39**:286-291

[312] Johnston IH, Duff J, Jacobson EE, Fagan E. Asymptomatic intracranial hypertension in disorders of CSF circulation in childhood-treated and untreated. Pediatric Neurosurgery. 2001;**34**:63-72

[313] Schoeman JF, Laubscher JA, Donald PR. Serial lumbar CSF pressure measurements and cranial computed tomographic findings in childhood tuberculous meningitis. Child's Nervous System. 2000;**16**:203-209

[314] Del Bigio MR, Kanfer JN, Zhang YW. Myelination delay in the cerebral white matter of immature rats with kaolin-induced hydrocephalus is reversible. Journal of Neuropathology and Experimental Neurology. 1997;**56**: 1053-1066

[315] De Vries LS, Liem KD, vanDijk K, Smit BJ, Sie L, Rademaker KJ, et al. Early versus late treatment of posthaemorrhagic ventricular dilatation: Results of a retrospective study from five neonatal intensive care units in The Netherlands. Acta Paediatrica. 2002;**91**: 212-217

[316] Xenos C, Sgouros S, Natarajan K, Walsh AR, Hockley A. Influence of shunt type on ventricular volume changes in children with hydrocephalus. Journal of Neurosurgery. 2003;**98**: 277-283

[317] Jain H, Natarajan K, Sgouros S. Influence of the shunt type in the difference in reduction of volume between the two lateral ventricles in shunted hydrocephalic children. Child's Nervous System. 2005;**21**:552-558

[318] Tuli S, O'Hayon B, Drake J, Clarke M, Kestle J. Change in ventricular size and effect of ventricular catheter placement in pediatric patients with shunted hydrocephalus. Neurosurgery. 1999;**45**:1329-1333

[319] Kolarovszki B, Žúbor P, Kolarovszká H, Benčo M, Richterová R, Maťašová K. The assessment of intracranial dynamics by transcranial Doppler sonography in perioperative

period in paediatric hydrocephalus. Archives of Gynecology and Obstetrics. 2013;**287**:229-238

[320] Kolarovszki B, Zibolen M, De Riggo J, Maťašová K, Šutovský J, Čiljak M, et al. Sledovanie dopplerovských parametrov prúdenia krvi v a. pericallosa u novorodencov s hydrocefalom pred drenážnym výkonom a po drenážnom výkone. Česko-slovenská pediatrie. 2006;**61**: 627-632

[321] Rennie JM. Neonatal Cerebral Ultrasound. Cambridge: Cambridge University Press; 1997. p. 242

[322] Cedzich C, Schramm J, Wenzel D. Reversible visual loss after shunt malfunction. Acta Neurochirurgica. 1990;**105**:121-123

[323] Newman NJ. Bilateral visual loss and disc edema in a 15 year-old girl. Survey of Ophthalmology. 1994;**38**: 365-370

[324] Gjerris F, Brogesen SE. Pathophysiology of CSF circulation. In: Crockard A, Hayward A, Hoff JT, editors. Neurosurgery. The Scientific Basis of Clinical Practice. Oxford: Blackwell Scientific; 1992. pp. 146-174

[325] da Silva PS, Suriano IC, Neto HM. Slitlike ventricle syndrome: A life-threatening presentation. Pediatric Emergency Care. 2009;**25**:674-676

[326] Eymann R, Schmitt M, Antes S, Shamdeen MG, Kiefer M. Dynamics of cerebrospinal fluid flow in slit ventricle syndrome. Acta Neurochirurgica. Supplement. 2012;**113**:181-186

[327] Teo C, Morris W. Slit ventricle syndrome. Contemporary Neurosurgery. 1999;**21**:1-4

[328] Gnanalingham KK, Lafuente D, Cheng D, Harkness W, Thompson D. Isolated diastasis of cranial sutures: Unusual presentation of a blocked shunt in an infant. Child's Nervous System. 2005;**21**:936-938

[329] McLaurin RL, Olivi A. Slit-ventricle syndrome: Review of 15 cases. Pediatric Neuroscience. 1987;**13**:118-124

[330] Sakamoto H, Kitano S. Reexpandability of the ventricular system of hydrocephalic children in the event of shunt occlusion. Child's Nervous System. 2006;**22**:517-522

[331] Hopf N, Grunert P, Fries G, Resch K, Perneczky A. Endoscopic third ventriculostomy: Outcome analysis of 100 consecutive cases. Neurosurgery. 1999;**44**:795-804

[332] Drake J. Editorial: Endoscopic third ventriculostomy. Journal of Neurosurgery. Pediatrics. 2012;**10**: 461-462

[333] Schmitt PJ, Jane JA Jr. A lesson in history: The evolution of endoscopic third ventriculostomy. Neurosurgical Focus. 2012;**33**:E11

[334] Buxton N, Turner B, Ramli N, Vloeberghs M. Changes in third ventricular size with neuroendoscopic third ventriculostomy: A blinded study. Journal of Neurology, Neurosurgery, and Psychiatry. 2002;**72**:385-387

[335] Kulkarni AV, Drake JM, Armstrong DC, Dirks PB. Imaging correlates of successful endoscopic third ventriculostomy. Journal of Neurosurgery. 2000;**92**:915-919

[336] Schwarz TH, Ho B, Prestigiacomo CJ, Bruce JN, Feldstein NA, Goodman RR. Ventricular volume following third ventriculostomy. Journal of Neurosurgery. 1999;**91**:20-25

[337] George E, Natarajan K, Sgouros S. Changes in ventricular volume in hydrocephalic children following

successful endoscopic third ventriculostomy. Child's Nervous System. 2004;**20**:834-838

[338] Cinalli G, Sainte-Rose C, Chumas P, Zerah M, Brunelle F, Lot G, et al. Failure of third ventriculostomy in the treatment of aqueductal stenosis in children. Journal of Neurosurgery. 1999; **90**:448-454

[339] Fukuhara T, Luciano MG, Kowalski RJ. Clinical features of third ventriculostomy failures classified by fenestration patency. Surgical Neurology. 2002;**58**:102-110

[340] Nowosławska E, Polis L, Kaniewska D, Mikołajczyk W, Krawczyk J, Szymański W, et al. Influence of neuroendoscopic third ventriculostomy on the size of ventricles in chronic hydrocephalus. Journal of Child Neurology. 2004;**19**:579-587

[341] Cohen AR. Endoscopic ventricular surgery. Pediatric Neurosurgery. 1993; **19**:127-134

[342] Schwarz TH, Yoon SS, Cutruzzola FW, Goodman RR. Third ventriculostomy: Post-operative ventricular size and outcome. Minimally Invasive Neurosurgery. 1996;**25**:57-63

[343] Di Rocco F, Grevent D, Drake JM, Boddaert N, Puget S, Roujeau T, et al. Changes in intracranial CSF distribution after ETV. Child's Nervous System. 2012;**28**:997-1002

[344] Papile L, Burnstein J, Burnstein R, Koffler H. Incidence and evolution of subependymal and intraventricular hemorrhage: A study of infants with birth weights less than 1,500 gm. The Journal of Pediatrics. 1978;**92**:529-534

[345] Robinson S. Neonatal posthemorrhagic hydrocephalus from prematurity: Pathophysiology and current treatment concepts. Journal of Neurosurgery. Pediatrics. 2012;**9**: 242-258

[346] Fulkerson DH, Vachhrajani S, Bohnstedt BN, Patel NB, Patel AJ, Fox BD, et al. Analysis of the risk of shunt failure or infection related to cerebrospinal fluid cell count, protein level, and glucose levels in low-birth-weight premature infants with posthemorrhagic hydrocephalus. Journal of Neurosurgery. Pediatrics. 2011;**7**:147-151

[347] Chittiboina P, Pasieka H, Sonig A, Bollam P, Notarianni C, Willis BK, et al. Posthemorrhagic hydrocephalus and shunts: What are the predictors of multiple revision surgeries? Journal of Neurosurgery. Pediatrics. 2013;**11**:37-42

[348] Willis B, Javalkar V, Vannemreddy P, Caldito G, Matsuyama J, Guthikonda B, et al. Ventricular reservoirs and ventriculoperitoneal shunts for premature infants with posthemorrhagic hydrocephalus: An institutional experience. Journal of Neurosurgery. Pediatrics. 2009;**3**: 94-100

[349] Horinek D, Cihar M, Tichy M. Current methods in the treatment of posthemorrhagic hydrocephalus in infants. Bratislavské Lekárske Listy. 2003;**104**:347-351

[350] Gurtner P, Bass T, Gudeman SK, Penix JO, Philput CB, Schinco FP. Surgical management of posthemorrhagic hydrocephalus in 22 low-birth-weight infants. Child's Nervous System. 1992;**8**:198-202

[351] Heep A, Engelskirchen R, Holschneider A, Groneck P. Primary intervention for posthemorrhagic hydrocephalus in very low birthweight infants by ventriculostomy. Child's Nervous System. 2001;**17**:47-51

[352] Yu B, Li S, Lin Z, Zhang N. Treatment of posthemorrhagic hydrocephalus in premature infants with subcutaneous reservoir drainage.

Pediatric Neurosurgery. 2009;**45**: 119-125

[353] Jian L, Hang-song S, Zheng-lang L, Li-sheng Y, Heng W, Nu Z. Implantation of Ommaya reservoir in extremely low weight premature infants with posthemorrhagic hydrocephalus: A cautious option. Child's Nervous System. 2012;**28**:1687-1691

[354] Wayenberg JL, Raftopoulos CH, Vermeylen D, Pardou A. Non-invasive measurement of intracranial pressure in the newborn and the infant: The Rotterdam teletransducer. Archives of Disease in Childhood. 1993;**69**:493-497

[355] Hunt RW, Warfield SK, Wang H, Kean M, Volpe JJ, Inder TE. Assessment of the impact of the removal of cerebrospinal fluid on cerebral tissue volumes by advanced volumetric 3D-MRI in posthaemorrhagic hydrocephalus in a premature infant. Journal of Neurology, Neurosurgery, and Psychiatry. 2003;**74**:658-660

[356] Boillat CA, Jones HC, Kaiser GL, Harris NG. Ultrastructural changes in the deep cortical pyramidal cells of infant rats with inherited hydrocephalus and the effect of shunt treatment. Experimental Neurology. 1997;**147**: 377-388

[357] Suda K, Sato K, Takeda N, Miyazawa T, Arai H. Early ventriculoperitoneal shunt—Effects on learning ability and synaptogenesis of the brain in congenitally hydrocephalus HTX rats. Child's Nervous System. 1994; **10**:19-23

[358] Marin-Padilla M. Developmental neuropathology and impact of perinatal brain damage. II: White matter lesions of the neocortex. Journal of Neuropathology & Experimental Neurology. 1997;**56**:219-235

[359] van Essen DC. A tension-based theory of morphogenesis and compact wiring in the central nervous system. Nature. 1997;**385**:313-318

[360] Dykes FD, Dunbar B, Lazarra A, Ahmann PA. Posthaemorrhagic hydrocephalus in high-risk preterm infants: Natural history, management, and long-term outcome. The Journal of Pediatrics. 1989;**114**:611-618

[361] Bassan H, Eshel R, Golan I, Kohelet D, Ben Sira L, Mandel D, et al., External Ventricular Drainage Study Investigators. Timing of external ventricular drainage and neurodevelopmental outcome in preterm infants with posthemorrhagic hydrocephalus. European Journal of Paediatric Neurology. 2012;**16**:662-670

[362] Lee IC, Lee HS, Su PH, Liao WJ, Hu JM, Chen JY. Posthemorrhagic hydrocephalus in newborns: Clinical characteristics and role of ventriculoperitoneal shunts. Pediatrics and Neonatology. 2009;**50**:26-32

[363] Wang KC, Lee JY, Kim SK, Phi JH, Cho BK. Fetal ventriculomegaly: Postnatal management. Child's Nervous System. 2011;**27**:1571-1573

[364] Ouahba J, Luton D, Vuillard E, Garel C, Gressens P, Blanc N, et al. Prenatal isolated mild ventriculomegaly: Outcome in 167 cases. BJOG. 2006;**113**: 1072-1079

[365] Peruzzi P, Corbitt RJ, Raffel C. Magnetic resonance imaging versus ultrasonography for the in utero evaluation of central nervous system anomalies. Journal of Neurosurgery. Pediatrics. 2010;**6**:340-345

[366] Bromley B, Frigoletto F, Benacerraf B. Mild fetal lateral cerebral ventriculomegaly: Clinical course and outcome. American Journal of Obstetrics and Gynecology. 2002;**164**:863-867

[367] Goldstein R, LaPidus A, Filly R, Cardoza J. Mild lateral cerebral

ventricular dilatation in utero: Clinical significance and prognosis. Radiology. 1990;**176**:237-242

[368] Kelly E, Allen V, Seaward G, Windrim R, Ryan G. Mild ventriculomegaly in the fetus, natural history, associated findings and outcome of isolated mild fetal ventriculomegaly: A literature review. Prenatal Diagnosis. 2001;**21**:697-700

[369] Den Hollander N, Vinkeesteijn A, Schmitz P, Castman-Berrevoets C, Wladimiroff J. Prenatally diagnosed fetal ventriculomegaly: Prognosis and outcome. Prenatal Diagnosis. 1998;**18**: 557-566

[370] Graham E, Duhl A, Ural S, Allen M, Blakemore K, Witter F. The degree of antenatal ventriculomegaly is related to pediatric neurological morbidity. The Journal of Maternal-Fetal Medicine. 2001;**10**:258-263

[371] Pilu G, Falco P, Gabrielli S, Perolo A, Sandri F, Bovicelli L. The clinical significance of fetal isolated cerebral borderline ventriculomegaly: Report of 31 cases and review of the literature. Ultrasound in Obstetrics & Gynecology. 1999;**14**:320-326

[372] Vergani P, Locatelli A, Strobelt N, Cavallone M, Ceruti P, Paterlini G, et al. Clinical outcome of mild fetal ventriculomegaly. American Journal of Obstetrics and Gynecology. 1998;**178**: 218-222

[373] Xie AL, Wang YH, Zhao YP, Ye Y, Chen XM, Jin HP, et al. Outcome and prognosis of isolated mild fetal ventriculomegaly in uterus. Zhonghua Fu Chan Ke Za Zhi. 2011;**46**:418-421 (abstract)

[374] Durfee S, Kim F, Benson C. Postnatal outcome of fetus with the prenatal diagnosis of asymmetric hydrocephalus. Journal of Ultrasound in Medicine. 2001;**20**:263-268

[375] Girard N, Ozanne A, Gire C, Millet V, Mancini J, Raybaud C. Conduite à tenir devant une dilatation ventriculaire. Archives de Pédiatrie. 2001;**8**(Suppl 2):436-437

[376] Lipitz S, Yagel S, Malinger G. Outcome of fetus with isolated borderline unilateral ventriculomegaly diagnosed at mid-gestation. Ultrasound in Obstetrics & Gynecology. 1998;**12**: 23-26

[377] Senat M, Bernard J, Schwarzler P, Britten J, Ville Y. Prenatal diagnosis and follow-up of 14 cases of unilateral ventriculomegaly. Ultrasound in Obstetrics & Gynecology. 1999;**14**: 327-332

[378] Haratz KK, Nardozza LM, de Oliveira PS, Rolo LC, Milani HJ, de Sá Barreto EQ, et al. Morphological evaluation of lateral ventricles of fetuses with ventriculomegaly by three-dimensional ultrasonography and magnetic resonance imaging: Correlation with etiology. Archives of Gynecology and Obstetrics. 2011;**284**: 331-336

[379] Minárik M. Niektoré otázniky pri transkraniálnej Dopplerovej sonografii u kriticky chorých detí. Czech-Slovak Pediatrics. 1999;**54**:697-699

[380] Bada HS, Miller JE, Menke JA, Menten TG, Bashiru M, Binstadt D, et al. Intracranial pressure and cerebral arterial pulsatile flow measurements in neonatal intraventricular haemorrhage. The Journal of Pediatrics. 1982;**100**: 291-296

[381] Hill A, Volpe JJ. Decrease in pulsatile flow in anterior cerebral arteries in infantile hydrocephalus. Pediatrics. 1982;**69**:4-7

[382] Fisher AQ, Livingstone JN II. Transcranial Doppler and real-time cranial sonography in neonatal

hydrocephalus. Journal of Child Neurology. 1989;**4**:64-69

[383] Aaslid R, Hubert P, Nornes H. Evaluation of cerebrovascular spasm with transcranial Doppler ultrasound. Journal of Neurosurgery. 1984;**60**:37-41

[384] De Assis MC, Machado HR. Transfontanellar Doppler ultrasound measurement of cerebral blood velocity before and after surgical treatment of hydrocephalus. Arquivos de Neuro-Psiquiatria. 1999;**57**(3B):827-835 (abstract)

[385] Nishimaki S, Yoda H, Seki K, Kawakami T, Akamatsu H, Iwasaki Y. Cerebral blood flow velocities in the anterior cerebral arteries and basilar artery in hydrocephalus before and after treatment. Surgical Neurology. 1990;**34**:373-377

[386] Saito M, Olby NJ, Spaulding K, Muñana K, Sharp NJ. Relationship among basilar artery resistance index, degree of ventriculomegaly, and clinical signs in hydrocephalic dogs. Veterinary Radiology & Ultrasound. 2003;**44**:687-694

[387] De Riggo J, Kolarovszki B, Richterová R, Kolarovszká H, Šutovský J, Ďurdík P. Measurement of the blood flow velocity in the pericallosal artery of children with hydrocephalus by transcranial Doppler ultrasonography—Preliminary results. Biomedical Papers. 2007;**151**:285-289

[388] Jindal A, Mahapatra AK. Correlation of ventricular size and transcranial Doppler findings before and after ventricular peritoneal shunt in patients with hydrocephalus: Prospective study of 35 patients. Journal of Neurology, Neurosurgery, and Psychiatry. 1998;**65**:269-271

[389] Kolarovszki B, Ďurdík P, Šutovský J, De Riggo J, Maťašová K, Čiljak M. Hodnotenie toku krvi a. pericallosa u novorodencov a dojčiat s hydrocefalom transkraniálnou dopplerovskou sonografiou. Diagnostika a terapia v pediatrii. Martin: Jesseniova lekárska fakulta UK; 2004. pp. 57-60

[390] Nadvi SS, Du Trevou MD, Vandelen JR, Gouws E. The use of TCD ultrasonography as a method of assessing ICP in hydrocephalic children. British Journal of Neurosurgery. 1994;**8**:573-577

[391] Erol FS, Yakar H, Artas H, Kaplan M, Kaman D. Investigating a correlation between the results of transcranial Doppler and the level of nerve growth factor in cerebrospinal fluid of hydrocephalic infants: Clinical study. Pediatric Neurosurgery. 2009;**45**:192-197

[392] van Bel F, van de Bor M, Baan J, Stijnen T, Ruys JH. Blood flow velocity pattern of the anterior cerebral arteries. Journal of Ultrasound in Medicine. 1988;**7**:553-559

[393] Alvisi C, Cerisoli M, Giulioni M, Monari P, Salvioli GP, Sandri F, et al. Evaluation of cerebral blood flow changes by transfontanelle Doppler ultrasound in infantile hydrocephalus. Child's Nervous System. 1985;**1**:244-247

[394] Weller RO, Shulman K. Infantile hydrocephalus: Clinical, histological and ultrastructural study of brain damage. Journal of Neurosurgery. 1972;**36**:255-265

[395] Wozniak M, McLone DG, Raimondi AJ. Micro and macrovascular changes as a direct cause of parenchymal destruction in congenital murine hydrocephalus. Journal of Neurosurgery. 1975;**43**:535-545

[396] Goh D, Minns RA, Hendry GM, Thambyayah M, Steers AJ. Cerebrovascular resistive index assessed by dupplex Doppler sonography and its relationship to intracranial pressure in

infantile hydrocephalus. Pediatric Radiology. 1992;**22**:246-250

[397] Goh D, Minns RA, Pye SD, Steers AJ. Cerebral blood flow velocity changes after ventricular taps and ventriculoperitoneal shunting. Child's Nervous System. 1991;7:452-457

[398] Iacopino DG, Zaccone C, Molina D, Todaro C, Tomasello F, Cardia E. Intraoperative monitoring of cerebral blood flow during ventricular shunting in hydrocephalic pediatric patients. Child's Nervous System. 1995;**11**: 483-486

[399] Cosan TE, Gucuyener D, Dundar E, Arslantas A, Vural M, Uzuner K, et al. Cerebral blood flow alterations in progressive communicating hydrocephalus: Transcranial Doppler assessment in an experimental model. Neurosurgical Focus. 2000;**9**:1-5

[400] Kolarovszki B, Šutovský J, Maťašová K, Čiljak M, De Riggo J, Abou Harb A. Význam transkraniálnej dopplerovskej sonografie v sledovaní hydrocefalu u novorodencov. Aktuality v neonatológii. Martin: Univerzita Komenského v Bratislave Jesseniova lekárska fakulta v Martine; 2004. pp. 56-59

[401] Quinn MW, Pople IK. MCA pulsatility in children with blocked CSF shunt. Journal of Neurology, Neurosurgery, and Psychiatry. 1992;**55**: 525-527

[402] Goh D, Minns RA. Intracranial pressure and cerebral arterial flow velocity indices in childhood hydrocephalus: Current review. Child's Nervous System. 1995;**11**:392-396

[403] Finn JP, Quinn MW, Hall-Craggs MA, Kendall BE. Impact of vessel distortion on transcranial Doppler velocity measurements: Correlation with magnetic resonance imaging. Journal of Neurosurgery. 1990;**73**: 572-575

[404] Anca IA. Hypoxic ischemic cerebral lesions of the newborn—Ultrasound diagnosis. Pictorial essay. Medical Ultrasonography. 2011;**13**: 314-319

[405] Schellinger D, Grant EG, Richardson JD. Cystic periventricular leukomalacia: Sonographic and CT findings. American Journal of Neuroradiology. 1984;**5**:439-445

[406] Fukuda S, Kato T, Kakita H, Yamada Y, Hussein HM, Kato I, et al. Hemodynamics of the cerebral arteries of infants with periventricular leukomalatia. Pediatrics. 2006;**117**:1-8

[407] Fukuda S, Mizuno K, Kakita H, Kato T, Hussein MH, Ito T, et al. Late circulatory dysfunction and decreased cerebral blood flow volume in infants with periventricular leukomalacia. Brain & Development. 2008;**30**:589-594

[408] Ilves P, Lintrop M, Talvik I, Muug K, Maipuu L, Metsvaht T. Low cerebral blood flow velocity and head circumference in infants with severe hypoxic ischemic encephalopathy and poor outcome. Acta Paediatrica. 2009; **98**:459-465

[409] Liu J, Cao HY, Huang XH, Wang Q. The pattern and early diagnostic value of Doppler ultrasound for neonatal hypoxic-ischemic encephalopathy. Journal of Tropical Pediatrics. 2007;**53**:351-354

[410] McCrea HJ, Ment LR. The diagnosis, management, and postnatal prevention of intraventricular hemorrhage in the preterm neonate. Clinics in Perinatology. 2008;**35**:777-792

[411] Miranda P. Intraventricular hemorrhage and posthemorrhagic hydrocephalus in the preterm infant. Minerva Pediatrica. 2010;**62**:79-89

[412] Tsitouras V, Sgouros S. Infantile posthemorrhagic hydrocephalus. Child's Nervous System. 2011;**27**:1595-1608

[413] Bashiru M, Russell J, Bada HS, Menke JA, Miles R, Summer D. Noninvasive detection of neonatal cerebrovascular disease. Bruit. 1980;**4**:42

[414] Ventriculomegaly Trial Group. Randomised trial of early tapping in neonatal posthaemorrhagic ventricular dilatation. Archives of Disease in Childhood;**65**:3-10

[415] Nishimaki S, Iwasaki Y, Akamatsu H. Cerebral blood flow velocity before and after cerebrospinal fluid drainage in infants with posthemorrhagic hydrocephalus. Journal of Ultrasound in Medicine. 2004;**23**:1315-1319

[416] Kempley ST, Gamsu HR. Changes in cerebral artery blood flow velocity after intermittent cerebrospinal fluid drainage. Archives of Disease in Childhood. 1993;**63**:74-76

[417] Quinn MW, Ando Y, Levene MI. Cerebral arterial and venous flow-velocity measurements in post-haemorrhagic ventricular dilatation and hydrocephalus. Developmental Medicine and Child Neurology. 1992;**34**: 863-869

[418] Maertzdorf WJ, Vles JS, Beuls E, Mulder ALM, Blanco CE. Intracranial pressure and cerebral blood flow velocity in preterm infants with posthaemorrhagic ventricular dilatation. Archives of Disease in Childhood. Fetal and Neonatal Edition. 2002;**87**:185-188

[419] Soul JS, Eichenwald E, Walter G, Volpe JJ, du Plessis AJ. CSF removal in infantile posthemorrhagic hydrocephalus results in significant improvement in cerebral hemodynamics. Pediatric Research. 2004;**55**:872-876

[420] van Alfen-van der Velden AA, Hopman JC, Klaessens JH, Feuth T, Sengers RC, Liem KD. Cerebral hemodynamics and oxygenation after serial CSF drainage in infants with PHVD. Brain and Development. 2007; **29**:623-629

[421] Kolarovszki B, Šutovský J, De Riggo J, Kolarovszká H. Indikácia drenážneho výkonu u novorodencov s hydrocefalom. Neonatologické zvesti. 2006;**10**:9-11

[422] Konje JC, Abrams KR, Taylor DJ. Normative values of Doppler velocimetry of five major fetal arteries as determined by color power angiography. Acta Obstetricia et Gynecologica Scandinavica. 2005;**84**: 230-237

[423] Su YM, Lv GR, Chen XK, Li SH, Lin HT. Ultrasound probe pressure but not maternal Valsalva maneuver alters Doppler parameters during fetal middle cerebral artery Doppler ultrasonography. Prenatal Diagnosis. 2010;**30**:1192-1197

[424] Zalel Y, Almog B, Seidman DS, Achiron R, Lidor A, Gamzu R. The resistance index in the fetal middle cerebral artery by gestational age and ventricle size in a normal population. Obstetrics and Gynecology. 2002;**100**: 1203-1207

[425] Malinger G, Svirsky R, Ben-Haroush A, Golan A, Bar J. Doppler-flow velocity indices in fetal middle cerebral artery in unilateral and bilateral mild ventriculomegaly. The Journal of Maternal-Fetal & Neonatal Medicine. 2011;**24**:506-510

[426] Mai R, Rempen A, Kristen P. Color flow mapping of the middle cerebral artery in 23 hydrocephalic fetuses. Archives of Gynecology and Obstetrics. 1995;**256**:155-158

[427] Voigt HJ, Deeg KH, Rupprecht T. Cerebral Doppler ultrasound in fetal

hydrocephalus. Zeitschrift für Geburtshilfe und Neonatologie. 1995; **199**:23-29

[428] Cavalheiro S, Moron AF, Almodin CG, Suriano IC, Hisaba V, Dastoli P, et al. Fetal hydrocephalus. Child's Nervous System. 2011;**27**: 1575-1583

[429] Cavalheiro S, Moron AF, Zymberg ST, Dastoli P. Fetal hydrocephalus—Prenatal treatment. Child's Nervous System. 2003;**19**: 561-573

[430] Pople IK. Doppler flow velocities in children with controlled hydrocephalus: Reference values for the diagnosis of blocked cerebrospinal fluid shunts. Child's Nervous System. 1992;**8**: 124-125

[431] Pople IK, Quinn MW, Bayston R, Hayward RD. The Doppler pulsatility index as a screening test for blocked ventriculo-peritoneal shunts. European Journal of Pediatric Surgery. 1991;**1** (Suppl):27-29

[432] Chadduck WM, Crabtree HM, Blankenship JB, Adametz J. Transcranial Doppler ultrasonography for the evaluation of shunt malfunction in pediatric patients. Child's Nervous System. 1991;**7**:27-30

[433] Vajda Z, Büki A, Vető F, Horváth Z, Sándor J, Dóczi T. Transcranial Doppler-determined pulsatility index in the evaluation of endoscopic third ventriculostomy (preliminary data). Acta Neurochirurgica. 1999;**141**:247-250

[434] Gera P, Gupta R, Sailukar M, Agarwal P, Parelkar S, Oak S. Role of transcranial Doppler sonography and pressure provacation test to evaluate the need for cerebrospinal fluid drainage in hydrocephalic children. Journal of Indian Association of Pediatric Surgeons. 2002;**7**:174-183

[435] Taylor GA. Effect of scanning pressure on the intracranial hemodynamics during transfontanellar duplex Doppler examinations. Radiology. 1992;**185**:763-766

[436] Kolarovszki B, Šutovský J, Ďurdík P, De Riggo J, Zubríková L, Kolarovszká H. Zmena vybraných parametrov dopplerovskej krivky a. pericallosa počas kompresívneho testu na prednej fontanele u dojčiat a batoliat s hydrocefalom pred drenážnym výkonom. In: Bánovčin a kol. Diagnostika a terapia v pediatrii. Martin: Univerzita Komenského Jesseniova lekárska fakulta; 2005. pp. 112-117

[437] Behrens A, Lenfeldt N, Ambarki K, Malm J, Eklund A, Koskinen LO. Transcranial Doppler pulsatility index: Not an accurate method to assess intracranial pressure. Neurosurgery. 2010;**66**:1050-1057

[438] Hanlo PW, Gooskens RH, Nijhuis IJ, Faber JA, Peters RJ, van Huffelen AC, et al. Value of transcranial Doppler indices in predincting raised ICP in infantile hydrocephalus. A study with review of literature. Child's Nervous System. 1995;**11**:595-603

[439] Hanlo PW, Peters RJ, Gooskens RH, Heethaar RM, Keunen RW, van Huffelen AC, et al. Monitoring intracranial dynamics by transcranial Doppler—A new Doppler index: Trans systolic time. Ultrasound in Medicine & Biology. 1995;**21**:613-621

[440] Leliefeld PH, Gooskens RH, Peters RJ, Tulleken CA, Kappelle LJ, Han KS, et al. New transcranial Doppler index in infants with hydrocephalus: Transsystolic time in clinical practice. Ultrasound in Medicine & Biology. 2009;**35**:1601-1606

[441] Leliefeld PH, Gooskens RH, Tulleken CA, Regli L, Uiterwaal CS, Han KS, et al. Noninvasive detection of the distinction between progressive and

compensated hydrocephalus in infants: Is it possible ? Journal of Neurosurgery. Pediatrics. 2010;**5**:562-568

[442] Galarza M, Lazareff JA. Transcranial Doppler in infantile cerebrospinal fluid disorders: Clinical validity. Neurological Research. 2004; **26**:409-413

[443] Rodríguez-Nuñez A, Somoza-Martín M, Gómez-Lado C, Eirís-Puñal J, Camiña-Darriba F, Rodríguez-Segade S, et al. Therapeutic criteria in communicating childhood hydrocephalus. Journal of Neurosurgical Sciences. 2008;**52**:17-21

[444] Archer LNJ, Evans DH. Doppler assessment of the neonatal cerebral circulation. In: Levene MI, Bennett MJ, Punt J, editors. Fetal and Neonatal Neurology and Neurosurgery: Churchill Livingstone; 1988. pp. 162-168

[445] Büdingen HJ, Freund HJ. Ultraschall-Diagnostik an hirnversorgenden Arterien. Deutsches Ärzteblatt. 1985;**82**:1843-1848

[446] Busija DW, Heistadt DD. Effects of activation of sympathetic nerves on cerebral blood flow during hypercapnia in cats and rabbits. The Journal of Physiology. 1984;**347**:35-45

[447] Cowan F. Acute effects of indomethacin on neonatal cerebral blood flow velocities. Early Human Development. 1987;**13**:343. (abstract)

[448] Diehl B, Stodieck SR, Diehl RR, Ringelstein EB. The photic driving EEG response and photoreactive cerebral blood flow in the posterior cerebral artery in controls and patients with epilepsy. Electroencephalography and Clinical Neurophysiology. 1998;**107**:8-12

[449] Dings J, Meixensberger J, Amschler J, Hamelbeck B, Roosen K. Brain tissue pO_2 in relation to cerebral perfusion pressure, TCD findings and TCD-CO_2 reactivity after severe head injury. Acta Neurochirurgica. 1996;**138**: 425-434

[450] Goldberg BB, Merton DA, Deane CR. An Atlas of Ultrasound Color Flow Imaging. London: Martin Dunitz; 1997. p. 290

[451] Gösling RG, King DH. Continuous wave ultrasound as an alternative and complement to X-ray in vascular examinations. In: Reneman RE, editor. Cardiovascular Applications of Ultrasound. Amsterdam: North-Holland; 1974. p. 282

[452] Greisen G, Johansen K, Ellison PH, Fredriksen PS, Mali J, Friis-Hansen B. Cerebral blood flow in the newborn infant: Comparison of Doppler ultrasound and 133 Xenon clearance. The Journal of Pediatrics. 1984;**104**: 411-418

[453] Jorch G. Intrazerebrale Blutströmung bei Früh- und Neugeborenen mit Fontanellen-Dopplerultraschall. Der Kinderarzt. 1987;**18**:9-13

[454] Jorch G, Jorch N. Failure of autoregulation of cerebral blood flow in neonates studied by pulsed Doppler ultrasound of the internal carotid artery. European Journal of Pediatrics. 1987; **146**:468-472

[455] Lundell BPW, Sonesson SE. Surgery or indomethacin? Ductus closure and cerebral blood flow. Early Human Development. 1987;**14**:141. (abstract)

[456] McAllister JP 2nd, Maugans TA, Shah VM, Truex RC Jr. Neuronal effects of experimentally induced hydrocephalus in newborn rats. Journal of Neurosurgery. 1985;**63**:776-783

[457] Owega A, Klingelhofer J, Sabri O, Kunert HJ, Albers M, Sass H. Cerebral

blood flow velocity in acute schizophrenic patients. A transcranial Doppler ultrasonography study. Stroke. 1998;**29**:1149-1154

[458] Perlman JM, Herscovitch P, Corriveau S, Raichle M, Volpe JJ. The relationship of cerebral blood flow velocity, determined by Doppler, to regional cerebral blood flow, determined by positron emission tomography. Pediatric Research. 1985; **19**:357

[459] Perlman JM, Hill A, Volpe JJ. The effect of patent ductus arteriosus on flow velocity in the anterior cerebral artery: Ductal steal in the premature newborn infant. The Journal of Pediatrics. 1981;**99**:767-771

[460] Perlman JM, Volpe JJ. Seizures in the preterm infant: Effects on cerebral flow velocity, intracranial pressure and arterial pressure. The Journal of Pediatrics. 1983;**102**:288-293

[461] Perlman JM, Volpe JJ. Episodes of apnea and bradycardia in preterm newborn: Impact on cerebral circulation. Pediatrics. 1985;**76**:333-338

[462] Pourcelot L. Applications cliniques de l'examen Doppler transcutané. In: Peronneau R, editor. Vélocimétrie ultrasonore Doppler. Paris: INSERM; 1975. p. 653

[463] Rahilly PM. Effects of sleep state and feeding on cranial blood flow of the human neonate. Archives of Disease in Childhood. 1988;**55**:265-270

[464] Roberts AE, McKinney WM. Blood flow velocities in three cerebral arteries in the same subject modulate during thinking. Journal of Neuroimaging. 1998;**8**:191-196

[465] Rosenkrantz TS, Oh W. Aminophyllin reduces cerebral blood flow velocity in low-birth-weight infants. American Journal of Diseases of Children. 1984;**138**:489-491

[466] Rubin R, Hochwald GM, Tiell M, Epstein F, Ghatak N, Wisniewski H. Hydrocephalus: III. Reconstitution of the cerebral cortical mantle following ventricular shunting. Surgical Neurology. 1976;**5**:179-183

[467] Rubin R, Hochwald GM, Tiell M, Liwnicz B, Epstein F. Reconstitution of the cerebral cortical mantle in shunt-corrected hydrocephalus. Developmental Medicine and Child Neurology. 1975;**35**:151-156

[468] Shortland DB, Gibson NA, Levene MI, Archer LNJ, Evans DH, Shaw DE. Patent ductus arteriosus and cerebral circulation in preterm infants. Developmental Medicine & Child Neurology. 1990;**32**:386-393

[469] Schwarz KH. Physik und Radiopioniere. Verlag Wetzikon; 1971. p. 170

[470] Vergesslich KA, Weninger M, Ponhold W, Simbruner G. Cerebral blood flow in newborn infants with and without mechanical ventilation. Pediatric Radiology. 1989;**19**:509-512

[471] Whitelaw A. Towards a molecular basis for intraventricular haemorrhage: Nitric oxide and impaired cerebral autoregulation. Acta Paediatrica. 2002; **91**:373-374

[472] Wright LL. Cerebral blood flow velocity in term newborn infants: Changes associated with ductal flow. Journal of Pediatrics. 1988;**112**:733-768